THE FIRST YEAR®

Celiac Disease

and Living Gluten-Free

Celiac Disease
and Living Gluten-Free

Jules E. Dowler Shepard

Da Capo
∞
LIFE
LONG

A MEMBER OF THE PERSEUS BOOKS GROUP

Set in 11 point Adobe Garamond by the Perseus Books Group.

Shepard, Jules E. Dowler.
    The first year : celiac disease and living gluten-free : an essential guide for the newly diagnosed / Jules E. Dowler Shepard. — 1st ed.
        p.   cm.
    Includes bibliographical references and index.
    ISBN 978-0-7382-1227-2 (alk. paper)
    1. Celiac disease—Popular works. 2. Gluten-free diet—Popular works.
I. Title.
RC862.C44S54 2008
616.3'99—dc22   2008033063

First Da Capo Press edition 2008

Published by Da Capo Press
A Member of the Perseus Books Group
www.dacapopress.com

Da Capo Press books are available at special discounts for bulk purchases in the United States by corporations, institutions, and other organizations. For more information, please contact the Special Markets Department at the Perseus Books Group, 2300 Chestnut Street, Suite 200, Philadelphia, PA 19103, or call (800) 810-4145, ext. 5000, or e-mail special.markets@perseusbooks.com.

20   19   18   17   16   15   14   13   12

To my mother and my grandmother, whose love for the kitchen and all things homemade instilled in me at an early age a passion for creating foods that bring joy to others.

Contents

Foreword

WHY ME? Why just me? And why, among all the diseases out there, did I get stuck with celiac disease?

These are among the most frequent questions that our newly diagnosed celiac patients ask themselves. Soon afterward, frustration, despair, denial, and depression sink in. People not afflicted by this condition may perceive these reactions disproportionate to what celiac disease is all about. But what really is celiac disease?

Celiac disease ("CD"), or gluten-sensitive enteropathy, is an immune-mediated, chronic condition. It targets the intestines so that they are not able to properly handle foodstuff anymore, leading to a wide range of clinical manifestations of variable severity. Besides the typical malabsorption symptoms (e.g., chronic diarrhea, weight loss, abdominal distension, etc.), CD can manifest itself in a previously unappreciated spectrum of symptoms that potentially can affect any organ system.

Indeed, because it is now more widely recognized, physicians have come to understand that fewer patients actually present with typical gastrointestinal symptoms. More frequent are patients with nonintestinal symptoms, such as anemia, joint pain, chronic fatigue, short stature, skin lesions, and neurological and behavioral problems (including peripheral neuropathy, epilepsy, dementia, schizophrenia, and seizure with intracranial calcifications). Because CD often presents in an atypical or even "silent" manner, many cases still remain undiagnosed. Such cases carry the risk of long-term complications in adolescence and adulthood, including osteoporosis, infertility, miscarriages, cancer, or the onset of other autoimmune diseases.

Until recently, the geographical distribution of CD was mostly restricted to Europe. New epidemiological studies, such as the one published in 2003 by the Center for Celiac Research at the University of Maryland, indicate that CD is common in other industrialized countries, such as the United States, Canada, and Australia as well as in many developing countries, suggesting that the "global village of CD" has a worldwide distribution. It appears that no continent on the planet is spared by the disease. It is projected that approximately 3 million Americans may be affected by CD, although only about one hundred thousand are diagnosed to date.

We are also learning that celiac disease is unique among autoimmune diseases in that we have identified its trigger is related to nutrition. Like other autoimmune diseases, celiac disease results from the interplay of a genetic predisposition and an environmental trigger. The particular trigger for celiac disease involves grains like wheat, rye, and barley, which contain a protein called gluten that is toxic for individuals with the condition. Thus, the fundamental cornerstone of treatment of celiac disease is a lifelong adherence to a strict gluten-free diet devoid of proteins from wheat, rye, barley, and related cereals. Gluten is, however, a common (and in many countries unlabeled) ingredient in the human diet, presenting a big challenge for celiac patients. Gluten-free products are not widely available and are typically far more expensive than their gluten-containing counterparts.

Despite the fact that a gluten-free diet is crucial for all celiac patients, these types of dietary hurdles have caused gluten-free compliance to be suboptimal in a strikingly large proportion of patients. It is indisputable that the main reason for failure of the gluten-free diet for celiac sufferers is related to lack of information, poor awareness among health care professionals and major confusion regarding what food products are safe and what are not. Once patients are correctly diagnosed, it is not unusual that their health care provider informs them of the need for a gluten-free diet but fails to provide their patients with any information on how to implement it. The reality is that going shopping for gluten-free products can be a daunting proposition involving hours of shopping, often resulting in only two to three items in your basket! Therefore, the idea of a "lifelong gluten-free diet" can translate into a sense of deprivation and powerlessness as to this permanent change in lifestyle.

Because food pervades nearly every social activity, each event needs to be carefully planned in advance to enjoy one of the most natural activities of humankind: eating. Shopping, cooking, avoiding cross-contamination, having a balanced and palatable diet . . . all become overwhelming enterprises, *until you read this book from Jules.* With her personal experience and a unique touch of humanity, Jules walks you through the major change in lifestyle that celiac disease imposes, going week by week, month by month, through the first year of embracing an entirely new diet. This book will take away the stress involved with simply understanding the rules of the game and fill in the blanks that your doctor many not have told you about. Jules's direct, personable, and friendly approach gives you a practical understanding of celiac disease, essential suggestions, and superb gluten-free recipes to help you eat healthy, well, and safely.

The First Year: Celiac Disease and Living Gluten-Free is truly a must for both beginners and "pros," both celiac and gluten intolerant—a book you want to have handy in your kitchen and by your bed so that you can go back to eating and socializing with a smile on your face.

—*Alessio Fasano, MD*

Dr. Fasano is the Medical Director of the Center for Celiac Research (CFCR) at the University of Maryland, which is recognized as a leader in the field of celiac disease. He is regarded as one of the foremost authorities worldwide on celiac disease, and his epidemiological studies in the United States have forever changed the preconception that celiac disease is a rare disorder in our county. The Center is located in Baltimore, Maryland, and houses a comprehensive, multidisciplinary program covering clinical care (for both children and adults), support services, education, and world-renown scientific research relating to celiac disease. The Center is responsible for many outstanding accomplishments, some of which are listed below:

1. Putting CD on the radar screen in the United States as a frequent, rather than a rare disease
2. Developing the Ttg blood screening test that is used now worldwide
3. Developing the genetic testing that is used worldwide
4. Educating health care professionals and the general public regarding celiac disease
5. Interfacing with Alba Therapeutics to accelerate the search for an alternative treatment/cure for CD.

For more information on the CFCR, please visit *www.celiaccenter.org* or *www.celiacwalk.org.*

Introduction

Celiac Disease? Celiac Sprue? Gluten-Free?

When I first heard those words, they were totally foreign to me. I had never heard of "celiac" (an autoimmune disorder characterized by inability to digest gluten) or "gluten" (a protein found in certain grains, including wheat), yet now I was forever linked to them. I was only twenty-nine when I was diagnosed and still thought I was immortal. The thought of being branded with an actual disease took my breath away.

On the one hand, I was in many ways relieved to know there was actually something diagnosably wrong with me. For the ten years prior, physicians had dubbed my numerous, unexplainable gastrointestinal problems as **irritable bowel syndrome** (IBS). As frustrating and unattractive as that sounded though, this new moniker—celiac disease—sounded even worse! And since at the time there were few resources for people with celiac, little did I know then how difficult it would be to learn to live a normal life with this new condition.

But I'm getting ahead of myself. My first year after learning I had celiac disease was truly a roller coaster of emotions and illness as I navigated that turbulent period on my own. No one was there to guide me over the many hurdles that presented themselves, one right after the other. As I look back on that time, now a decade ago, I want nothing more than to save others from having such a rough time of it. If I had only had someone to point me in the right direction upon my diagnosis: to tell me the questions to ask, the stores where I could shop, the foods I could eat, and what I could expect to experience, I literally would have been spared years of lonely trial and error. My hope is that this book will put you on the fast track to a happy and healthy gluten-free life.

My Story

Growing up, I was the typical girl-child whose favorite toy was her Easy-Bake Oven. Luckily, my indulgent mother and grandmother let me "help" them often in the kitchen, and I acquired from an early age a love and respect for food as a way of joyously bringing people together.

As I grew older, my Southern upbringing taught me food was a conduit for socializing. My mother and I baked goodies at the holidays to share with friends and neighbors, wrapping them with decorative bows and presenting them on doorsteps, at school, at church, and at parties. We were also renowned for our sugar cookies, made in every color and shape to celebrate the seasons.

I carried these traditions with me as I went off on my own to college and then to graduate school. I quickly became popular in the dorm for breaking the rules by firing up my toaster oven to bake loads of chocolate chip cookies to share. In law school, baking became a serious stress reliever for me. I found myself more and more frequently baking in the wee hours of the morning to unwind from hours of studying. I shared my muffin, bread, and cake experiments with all my friends because I made far too many for my roommate and I to eat ourselves. Soon, the school café invited me to sell my baked goods there, presumably because their business was suffering from the steady supply of my free food! Friends would call on me for advice on baking and nutrition, and I was always part of the group having potluck dinners.

I remember the very day I first became sick. It was the last day of spring break and I enjoyed a nice dinner of shrimp scampi and pasta with my boyfriend and his parents at the beach. The next day, I was sick with every embarrassing and uncomfortable tummy trouble I could imagine, the whole drive home from Florida to North Carolina. And from that point forward, I never got better. I did not associate my sickness with eating because I never noticed a link between what I ate—foods I had previously enjoyed my whole life—and subsequently becoming ill. I had been a vegetarian since the age of sixteen, so my college diet was mostly cheap pizza, bagels, pasta, cereal, and fruit (with the exception of the latter, all major gluten offenders).

Faced with constant abdominal bloating and pain, I started seeing doctor after doctor, who ran every even more embarrassing test I could imagine. But the gastroenterologists had no solutions. I recall them consistently urging me to eat more fiber—which I did, by eating more breads and cereals like All-Bran and Shredded Wheat. (I was that annoying student who munched on the bag of dry Frosted Mini-Wheats all through the 8 a.m. class!) Never did anyone realize that maybe those foods were precisely what were causing my discomfort.

By the time I was a stressed-out prosecuting attorney, I had been treated for over ten years by specialists in the five states in which I'd lived, and I had only steadily gotten worse. The diagnosis I had consistently received, IBS, was the physical equivalent of everyone's throwing their hands up in frustration and guessing. Although IBS is a real condition many are indeed afflicted with, with me it was simply a speculation—they had no idea what was wrong with me. They prescribed antispasmodic medications, less stress, and of course even more gluten-filled fiber.

When I met my sixth gastroenterologist in 1999, my chief complaint was that I was forced to spend nearly every morning in the basement of the local courthouse in a room the size of a walk-in closet with a dozen police officers, a half-dozen public defenders and defense attorneys, a stray magistrate or two, and a victim advocate . . . and my bloated belly was causing me, not only pain, but bad gas! The awkwardness of it was matched only by the discomfort it caused me. I was desperate for something, anything, to make it better!

When this latest doctor asked about my diet, I was dismissive because I had been down this road so many fruitless times before. He persisted, though, and suggested that I should be tested for something called "celiac sprue." Of course, I had never heard of this dreaded condition and was certain I didn't have it—I must just need more fiber, right? Ultimately, I allowed him to perform an upper endoscopy (I was anaesthetized and a scope was placed down my throat and into my upper intestinal tract, where they proceeded to biopsy tissue samples). After the test, the doctor showed me the pictures and told me frankly that he did not even need the tissue samples because he could tell from simply looking at my intestines that I had celiac disease. Apparently, what to me looked from the pictures like a healthy, smooth, bright pink tube, should have been a paler, wider tube full of fingerlike villi. I presented the classic auto-immune response to gluten . . . and I had never even heard of gluten!

So, what was I to do now that I knew the root of all my ailments? Well, my gastroenterologist certainly didn't know. He very astutely determined that I had celiac disease and was kind enough to tell me to never eat gluten again, but he had no idea as to how I should do that, exactly. So, I walked out of his office with a real diagnosis, feeling more confused, and even more frustrated than I had been when I walked in thinking I simply had an out-of-control bout with IBS. Why couldn't I have something that just needed a pill? How did I end up with something that meant radically changing my diet and my life forever?

I was a month away from my wedding day, so I felt even more pressure. I searched the Internet, the library, and the brains of anyone I could find who might be able to help me avoid this thing called gluten. The best I could do was to eat Peppermint Patties and rice cakes until I could figure out what to do. My fiancé thoughtfully went out and bought several jumbo boxes of Rice Krispies cereal, which we were both very excited about until we discovered that the malt flavoring in the cereal contained gluten. Poor thing, he had to eat Rice Krispies for months! (On the positive side, I was glad that I went hard-core gluten-free that month, because I lost a dress size from not being bloated anymore.)

We couldn't change the wedding menu in such a short time, and I wouldn't have known what to tell the caterer to make in the alternative any-way, so I cheated at the reception and even drank beer. I paid for it later, of course, but at that time I did not understand (beyond the immediate conse-quences) the implications of ingesting gluten.

There were certainly times in the beginning that I wished I could cheat again with blissful ignorance of the long-term consequences. Unfortunately, though, my body would not let me get off so easily, and I soon learned that even small amounts of gluten took their toll. Thankfully, I now sit in a posi-tion of experienced wisdom and comfortable understanding that comes from years of experimentation and education. It is possible to regain the social life I had before, to bake for my friends and family, to share meals and parties to-gether again, to travel internationally, and to live in a nearly normal way. I traveled a long road to get to this point, however, and I hope that the trials and errors shared with you in this book will guide you to a comfortable place much faster!

Cooking Gluten-Free

My early experiments with gluten-free cooking were, in a word, disastrous. My new husband at first tried to eat them and be kind, but it didn't take long for him to simply take a pass on anything I made that was gluten-free. In many ways I felt worse for him than for myself, as he had not really signed on for this life! When we met and while we dated, I cooked real meals and they were really good. I baked all the time and he was spoiled by having yummy homemade treats around. Suddenly, though, I was no longer making palatable food at home and he felt guilty eating in front of me at restaurants when I could find nothing on the menu that was safe for me.

The situation was getting desperate. I finally caved and began making real food again, but only he or our guests could eat it. I was relegated to eating the dry, gritty, hard, and often overly sweet food that was available gluten-free. Through research and comparison, I found that the gluten-free recipes and premade food used an excess of sweeteners in an attempt to mask the otherwise unpleasant flavors and consistencies of the gluten-free ingredients. These foods were also heavy on rice flour as a substitute for wheat flours. I learned that rice flour tends to make foods bulky and gritty if it is not balanced by other finer starches. Initially, I was too frustrated to experiment with recipes to overcome these problems; I simply stopped cooking altogether.

But more than just missing the food (and longing to lick the bowl again!), I missed exercising that portion of my personality that yearned to create, experiment, and bake foods, and I missed bringing pleasure to others through my cooking. At the time, I felt that a chunk of my life had been snatched away by my diagnosis with celiac. It was only when I learned that I was pregnant though, that I realized *good* gluten-free cooking was something I simply had to master for myself and for my family. With renewed vigor, I began in earnest to experiment with recipes, gluten-free flours, and other alternative ingredients to find palatable and nutritional options.

My husband adopted the new role of barometer in my baking process. He began to taste my food again and to critique it—sometimes taking a second helping, often not. I tried everything: pizza, pies, cakes, cookies, casseroles, pasta. There were some raw moments, such as when I furiously grabbed yet another failed and crumbly pie crust and hurled it into the trash can, swearing that I would never bake another gluten-free pastry again. Some days I think my husband was simply afraid to ask how my experiments had gone! One day, though, after my playing around with a mixture of five flours to create a scone recipe, he tasted one on his way out the door and actually came back inside to grab a handful more to take with him. I jumped for joy. I had done it—I had come up with a gluten-free recipe that was good enough for someone without celiac disease to *choose* to have seconds or thirds!

From that recipe, I was able to devise my base gluten-free flour mixture, Nearly Normal All-Purpose Flour. Once I had a successful flour mix, I found that I could use it with success to replace wheat flour in almost any recipe. The door was open and I ran through it! My life had changed. Friends and family began to eat my food unknowingly, thinking that I had made something else gluten-free for myself to eat instead. When they asked for leftovers and recipes, I felt my old self returning and rose to the challenge of baking gluten-free for everyone.

Having achieved success only through years of experimentation and baking nearly every day, I appreciate that not all people can or should go through those trials themselves once they are diagnosed. I published a cookbook, *Nearly Normal Cooking for Gluten-Free Eating,* so that others may have a variety of tried-and-true (and safe) recipes they could proudly serve. Many portions of this book are also dedicated to sharing my tips for successful gluten-free cooking and feature recipes to begin your new life ahead.

I now teach classes on gluten-free cooking, and through those opportunities as well as through e-mails from celiacs and those who are gluten-intolerant, I hear from so many others who share in the frustrations of cooking and eating gluten-free. I know that it is not always easy or fun or tasty, but I also know that it is possible to make it such. I hope that you will take away from this book a recognition of the true need for celiacs to abide by a strict gluten-free diet, an understanding of how to cook successfully with gluten-free flours, and the confidence to go back out into the world safely and successfully in spite of your diagnosis. I will not prescribe a course of action for you in this book, as everyone's experiences with the disease are somewhat unique; however, these general guidelines should assist you in making choices for your life ahead.

Necessity is truly the mother of invention, so I encourage you, too, to experiment in your own kitchen and in your life to see if it opens new doors for you.

A Journey to Good Health

My cookbook and Web sites, www.NearlyNormalCooking.com and www
.NearlyNormalKitchen.com, are wonderful ways of communicating with others around the world who share this dining disorder. They also have introduced me to so many celiacs with their own stories of challenge and success
that I recognized the need to convey their earned wisdom as well. Only
through sharing our collective experiences can we spare the newly diagnosed
from our collective mistakes. In writing this book, I hope to hold the hands of
millions of those who will be diagnosed with celiac disease in the coming
years. Researchers believe 1 out of every 133 people has celiac, but only a
small percentage of those are yet aware that they have the disease. As modern
medicine advances and these suffers are made aware of their celiac diagnosis,
they will find themselves needing the support and expertise of those who have
already begun the journey of living life with celiac disease. I hope that this
book provides the guidance and understanding that you seek as you embark
on a new life, and that through it, you may live nearly normally despite celiac
disease. I wish you all the best on your personal journey to good health.

learning

What Is Celiac Disease (in Plain English)?

CELIAC DISEASE[1] (also known as **celiac sprue**, cœliac disease, nontropical sprue, or gluten-sensitive enteropathy) is a chronic and permanent sensitivity to the food protein **gluten**, found in the grains wheat, barley, and rye. Developing the disease requires three things: a genetic predisposition, exposure to gluten through digestion, and a trigger to start this atypical immune system response. It can occur in people of all ages once they have been exposed to gluten and is the most common genetic disorder in North America and Europe, although it is found in populations all over the world.

---

1. There has been some dispute over what to call this disease and over what to call a person who has it. Celiac sprue was the early name for the battery of symptoms we now recognize as celiac disease. The term *cœliac* or *celiac* is the Greek word for abdominal region; *sprue* refers to a disease of the small intestine. Thus, some feel it is incorrect to call this autoimmune disease simply "celiac." I will avoid arguing over linguistic semantics and throughout this book will simply refer to the disease as "celiac disease" or "CD" and to a diagnosed individual as "a celiac." Right or wrong, this terminology has become customary.

By now you probably already know that celiac disease (CD) is classified as an **autoimmune disease**, which simply means that the body attacks *itself* in an inappropriate immune system reaction. In CD, the reaction is caused specifically by exposure to **gliadin**, a protein of the food molecule gluten found in wheat, barley, and rye; in most all other autoimmune diseases, the catalyst for starting the inappropriate reaction in the body is not yet known.

Looking further into the actual "celiac reaction" requires a review of the small intestines. In a normal, healthy person, the small intestine is lined with shag carpet–like projections of tissue called **villi**, which absorb valuable nutrients into the bloodstream and block the absorption of other molecules. In a person with celiac disease, though, the intestinal linings are abnormally permeable, allowing some molecules like gluten to be absorbed through the gut. This leakage through the intestines initiates an immune assault that causes an inflammatory reaction and damages the villi that have absorbed it.

Through repeated absorption and ensuing damage, these villi are ultimately blunted and flattened, destroying the body's ability to properly absorb food (called "**villous atrophy**"). The result: your intestines can no longer efficiently or effectively absorb *any* nutrients from your food, not just gluten. This damage begins a chain reaction in the body that you may or may not notice, depending on how long your body has manifested this active celiac reaction and on your unique symptomology. The only treatment or prevention of this effect in a person with celiac disease is to adhere to a lifelong gluten-free diet. There is no magic pill.

Celiac, Wheat Allergy, and Gluten Intolerance: What's the Difference?

Other very different conditions, such as gluten intolerance and wheat allergy, at times mimic celiac disease symptoms and are also treated with a gluten-free diet. However, these conditions are all quite different from celiac disease, and it is important to accurately diagnose which condition is causing your distress.

An allergy to wheat is actually very different from celiac disease, in that it is not an autoimmune disorder at all, but the body's mistaken immune system response to a harmless food protein. The body creates antibodies to this protein that attach themselves to the food molecule and then cause other cells to attack by releasing histamines. The body's attack may produce a variety of symptoms, often unique to the individual. These symptoms are often rapid and may be severe, ranging from a skin rash to gastrointestinal distress, swelling, migraines, or even difficulty breathing. Once the allergen is removed from the body or antihistamines are successfully administered, the body is not compromised in the long term as it is for those who have celiac disease and are exposed to gluten.

Gluten intolerance is another condition that requires adherence to a gluten-free diet but does not rise to the level of an autoimmune disease. Food intolerances occur when the body is incapable of metabolizing certain foods, typically because it lacks certain enzymes necessary to break down particular food components. Those with gluten intolerance often have the same overt symptoms as those with CD, but they test negative for celiac disease by bloodwork and endoscopy. They learn through trial and error that gluten is the culprit for their uncomfortable symptoms and, once they adopt a gluten-free diet, live an otherwise normal healthy life.

As discussed, celiac disease is an autoimmune condition, whereby the body's immune system attacks its own intestinal tissue in an inappropriate response to eating gluten. The damage caused by untreated celiac disease can lead to **malabsorption** of food, which in turn can cause nutritional deficiencies, anemia, rickets, kidney stones, osteomalacia, and osteoporosis. Unlike celiac disease, food intolerances and allergies do not typically cause severe intestinal damage and, therefore, do not generally lead to nutritional deficiencies.

As an autoimmune disorder, celiac disease necessarily involves the activation of the immune system. Autoimmune diseases such as celiac also increase the likelihood that the patient may contract other autoimmune conditions, such as lupus, thyroid disease, type 1 diabetes, liver diseases, or joint diseases, including rheumatoid arthritis. Celiacs, as opposed to those who suffer from food allergies and intolerances, even have an elevated risk of developing gastrointestinal cancers like lymphomas.[2] By contrast, those who suffer from wheat allergy or gluten intolerance, neither of which is an immune system response, are not at any increased risk of developing an autoimmune condition or cancer as a result of their allergy or intolerance.

---

2. Mayo Clinic, "Digestive System: Celiac Disease," MayoClinic.com. http://www.mayoclinic.com/health/celiac-disease/DS00319/DSECTION=7.

Thus, it is crucial to understand the root cause of your problems with gluten. If you have CD, your physician must monitor your nutritional deficiencies and look for any signs of other autoimmune diseases or gastrointestinal cancers, in particular. Celiac disease is hereditary as well, so knowing whether or not you have the condition will instruct you and your family members as to whether they should be tested to protect their health.

Celiac Disease vs. Food Allergies and Intolerances

Celiac Disease	Wheat/Gluten Allergy or Intolerance
may cause gastrointestinal symptoms	may cause gastrointestinal symptoms
autoimmune condition	not autoimmune related
causes intestinal damage	does not cause intestinal damage
will cause malabsorption of food	no direct link to malabsorption
will cause nutritional deficiencies	no direct link to nutritional deficiencies
increases risk of other autoimmune diseases	no increased risk of autoimmune disease
elevated risk of gastrointestinal cancers	no elevated risk of cancer
may cause neurological damage	no link to neurological damage
hereditary	not clearly hereditary
treated with gluten-free diet	treated with gluten-free diet

IN A SENTENCE

Celiac disease is not a food allergy/intolerance but an autoimmune disorder whereby the body inappropriately absorbs and attacks the food protein gliadin found in gluten, causing serious damage to the upper intestinal tract of a person afflicted with the disease and initiating a negative physiological chain reaction.

living

How Do You Know If You Have Celiac Disease?

MANY PEOPLE have suffered through years of unexplained symptoms that could actually be attributed to celiac disease. Because an unhealthy intestinal tract can affect virtually any other system in the body, celiac symptoms are often difficult to distinguish from the symptoms of many other conditions. A person may have an otherwise unexplained history of migraines, another of arthritis, and still another of chronic fatigue or thyroid problems, and yet all may later discover the root cause has been untreated celiac disease. A holistic approach to health is thus the best way to initially evaluate the potential for celiac or other conditions.

Fortunately, extremely accurate blood tests combined with **endoscopic biopsy** can ultimately yield a firm, positive diagnosis, but determining whether celiac could be the root of your particular problems is the first step. A partial list of potential symptoms of celiac disease is provided on the next page, and is more thoroughly discussed in this chapter. The sheer number of potential symptoms is amazing to see, but look closely at the enormous variation in the celiac symptoms as well. These symptoms can occur individually, in combination, sporadically, or constantly. Also bear in mind that the majority of those with undiagnosed celiac disease actually suffer no overt symptoms, although they still risk suffering its complications. This phenomenon is referred to as the "**Celiac Iceberg**," as the majority of celiacs are still under the surface, so to speak, since they are asymptomatic. (Go to my Web site to view a diagram of the celiac iceberg. http://NearlyNormalCooking .com/FY/)

Potential Celiac Symptoms

○ anemia (low hemoglobin or hematocrit)
○ autoimmune disorders such as rheumatoid arthritis and lupus
○ behavioral changes (can include depression, irritability, failure to concentrate)
○ bloating and gas or abdominal distention
○ bone or joint pain
○ changes in appetite
○ chronic diarrhea
○ colitis
○ collagen vascular disease
○ constipation
○ dermatitis herpetiformis (burning, itchy, and blistering skin rash)
○ delayed growth in children and delayed onset of puberty
○ dizziness
○ easy bruising
○ failure to thrive in infancy
○ fatigue and lethargy
○ fibromyalgia
○ hair loss
○ headaches
○ hypoglycemia (low blood sugar)
○ hyposplenism (underactive spleen)
○ increased risk of infections
○ infertility and miscarriage
○ iron deficiency
○ irregular or speedy heartbeat
○ lactose intolerance
○ liver disease

- ○ lupus
- ○ lymphoma (cancer of the lymph glands)
- ○ malnutrition
- ○ missed menstrual periods
- ○ mental fogginess
- ○ muscle cramps
- ○ nausea and/or vomiting
- ○ neurological problems (including schizophrenia, ataxia, and epilepsy)
- ○ nosebleeds
- ○ osteoporosis or osteopenia
- ○ pale, foul-smelling, bulky, and/or fatty stools that float
- ○ pale skin
- ○ seizures
- ○ short stature
- ○ shortness of breath
- ○ Sjögren's syndrome
- ○ some intestinal cancers
- ○ thyroid disease (hyper- or hypothyroidism)
- ○ tingling or numbness in the hands and feet
- ○ tooth discoloration or dental enamel defects/loss
- ○ type 1 diabetes
- ○ ulcers inside the mouth (aphthous ulcers)
- ○ vitamin or mineral deficiency
- ○ weight loss/gain

Underlying all of these potential symptoms is the damage to the small intestine and resulting nutrient, carbohydrate, and fat absorption issues. Untreated celiac disease ultimately leads to malnutrition, which in turn causes a host of other health problems. For example, malabsorption of calcium and vitamin D and K can cause osteopenia (reduced mineral content in bones) or even osteoporosis (progressive bone thinning and weakening). Miscarriage and birth defects can arise due to poor nutrient absorption and other resulting problems. Failure to thrive in infancy and short stature and delayed development in children occur when there is a serious lack of nutrition. Anemia results from iron malabsorption or from folic acid and vitamin B_{12} deficiencies. Further complications include developing other autoimmune diseases, thyroid problems, reproductive health issues, and even cancer, which can result if celiac disease is ignored or left untreated.[3]

It is crucial that the medical community understand and aggressively test for active celiac disease to prevent further physical complications from arising. CD is often misdiagnosed as irritable bowel syndrome (IBS), anemia, chronic fatigue syndrome, intestinal infection, and even Crohn's disease. If any of these diagnoses is suspected, or unexplained symptoms such as those listed in this chapter present themselves, ask your doctor to test you for celiac disease, to rule out that it is the root cause. A recent multicenter study demonstrated that when primary care physicians offer to test any patient exhibiting any of the myriad symptoms of celiac disease, the diagnostic rate increases thirty-two- to forty-three-fold! Early diagnosis is crucial to preventing serious consequences from untreated celiac disease, such as anemia, infertility, osteoporosis, and even cancer.[4]

IN A SENTENCE

> *Celiac disease may be disguised under many layers or confusing symptoms, so it is important to view your own symptoms holistically, to give your doctor the total picture of your health.*

---

3. Mayo Clinic, "Digestive System: Celiac Disease," MayoClinic.com. http://www.mayo clinic.com/health/celiac-disease/DS00319/DSECTION=7.

4. C. Catassi et al., "Detection of Celiac Disease in Primary Care: A Multicenter Case-Finding Study in North America," *American Journal of Gastroenterology* 102 (2007): 1454–60.

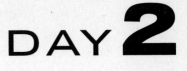
Taking the Tests

IF YOU believe that you have any of the symptoms of celiac disease, or if your physician feels that there is a chance you may have the condition, specific testing is needed. Since many of these symptoms are not exclusive to CD, it is important to be tested to rule out or confirm a diagnosis of celiac. It is also important that before any testing is undertaken, you continue to eat gluten. It may sound counterproductive to continue to eat gluten before you are tested if you suspect that gluten is making you sick, yet it is essential to a positive diagnosis via blood test or endoscopy. Both tests are looking for your body's reaction to gluten, to medically confirm a diagnosis of celiac disease. It follows that if you stop eating gluten, your body will stop reacting to gluten and will begin to heal itself, thus potentially masking the disease.

Blood Tests

The first testing will likely be in the form of a simple blood test ordered by your doctor. Blood tests have recently become very accurate, very quick, and far less expensive than they used to be (most insurance plans will cover this routine procedure, but you may want to confirm coverage with your plan administrator prior to undergoing any lab testing).

Your doctor will order a **celiac panel** of tests to discern whether you carry a higher-than-normal level of certain antibodies in your blood. Antibodies are the normal immune system's response to threatening substances within the body; however, the presence of particular antibodies in certain numbers can help to show whether your body is exhibiting a celiac reaction.

The celiac panel used in screening for the disease usually tests for antiendomysial antibody (IgA), antitissue transglutaminase (IgA), antigliadin (IgA and IgG), and total serum IgA against particular antigens in the small bowel, such as tissue transglutaminase (tTG).[1]

Genetic Tests

You may choose to have genetic testing to determine if you or your family members carry the **HLA typing** that nearly all celiacs have (these genes are called DQ2 and DQ8); if you do not carry this HLA typing, it is highly unlikely that you have or will ever develop active celiac disease.[2] Since genes are inherited through families, some celiacs opt to have their children tested genetically to prevent their undergoing later lab testing for active celiac disease. However, it is important to understand that this testing will not indicate whether one has active celiac disease and it is often not covered by insurance plans.

Endoscopy

Whether or not the blood tests indicate celiac disease, your doctor may want to perform a small bowel biopsy, or endoscopy. It is a simple and painless outpatient procedure but requires some level of anesthesia. A tube is inserted into your mouth and passed down into the small intestines, where pictures are taken of portions of the walls of the intestinal tract and small biopsy samples are removed for study in a lab. The physician will obtain several samples from different sections of your bowel to reduce the likelihood of a false negative result. The photos taken of the intestinal tract will aid in diagnosis, as the presence of certain visual

---

1. American Celiac Disease Alliance, http://americanceliac.org/diagnosis.htm.

2. Dietary proteins in gluten interact with these HLA molecules and cause abnormal mucosal immune responses that induce tissue damage. National Institutes of Health Consensus Development Conference Final Statement: Celiac Disease (August 9, 2004).

indicators like a scalloping of the folds in the small bowel and blunted villi may contribute to the accurate diagnosis of celiac disease. (Go to my Web site to view these historical features. http://NearlyNormalCooking.com/FYI/)

Promising studies at the Mayo Clinic may lead to future use of capsule endoscopy to detect and diagnose celiac disease and measure intestinal healing following treatment with a gluten-free diet. This type of endoscopy is even less traumatic to patients, as it simply requires a patient to swallow a vitamin-size capsule that contains a miniature color video camera, light, battery, and transmitter. The capsule moves through the small intestine in approximately eight hours and is passed by the patient in a normal bowel movement. The information it transmits is received and digitally recorded by a device worn by the patient. The capsule allows a physician to view all thirty feet of the small intestine, rather than just the first one or two feet that can been seen with traditional endoscopy.[3]

Skin Biopsy

If you have an itchy, blistering, and painful skin rash (usually around the elbows, knees, and buttocks), your doctor will follow a different course. The blood tests may be ordered but, rather than performing an endoscopy, the rash itself is biopsied for suspected **dermatitis herpetiformis** ("DH"). (Go to my Web site to view a photograph of DH. http://NearlyNormalCooking.com/FYI/)

If the antibody and skin biopsy are both positive for celiac disease, the intestinal biopsy is not necessary to confirm a diagnosis, as only around 20 percent of people who have DH also have the intestinal symptoms of CD. Regardless of the presence or absence of intestinal symptoms, those with confirmed DH diagnoses also must commit to a lifelong adherence to a gluten-free diet. Medications may be administered to aid in controlling the skin symptoms, but those medications alone do not control celiac disease.

IN A SENTENCE

> *Numerous tests are now widely available to help confirm a diagnosis of celiac disease, and it is likely that your doctor will want to administer both blood tests and a confirmatory endoscopic biopsy before making a firm diagnosis.*

---

3. Mayo Clinic, "Mayo Clinic Finds Capsule Endoscopy Can Detect Intestinal Damage Caused by Celiac Disease: Study Shows Extent of Intestinal Damage Does Not Explain Patients' Symptoms," http://www.mayoclinic.org/news2008-rst/4669.html (February 27, 2008).

living

The Importance of Being Tested

THE GOOD news is that many more physicians are aware of celiac disease and its symptoms than ever before. However, doctors can't know everything, and some are still unaware of the range of symptoms and that a simple blood test exists to find their source. Until very recently, medical schools did not spend much time on celiac disease, as it was considered to be so rare. There are no drugs to treat or cure it, so pharmaceutical companies are not educating the practicing doctors on the disease, either. Many specialists do not think of CD when presented with symptoms outside of the digestive system.

I have heard countless stories from students in my gluten-free cooking classes who demanded that their physicians test them for celiac disease when the doctors themselves have assured them that they did not have it—and as it turned out, they did.

One consulting client of mine recounted a story of being severely chastised by her longtime internist when she wondered aloud if her thyroid disease, intermittent severe digestive problems, migraines, and fatigue could be celiac disease. (Her cousin had been diagnosed, so she learned about the possible symptoms through him.) Her physician condescendingly told her that she did not have CD and that he would not order the tests because the condition is so rare, the tests are so expensive, and the lab work is not covered by insurance! All of these assumptions are false, and he was misinformed. Another client was tested only after she insisted that her gynecologist order the celiac panel because of her thyroid problems, sudden weight gain, hair loss, and digestive troubles. Her gynecologist was leery, though, and told her that she (the doctor) would have to look up celiac disease in her medical books because out of all of her thousands of patients, none of them had ever had CD! Statistically speaking, that fact is impossible, since researchers are now finding that 1 out of every 133 people has it. No wonder 95–97 percent of celiacs have still not been diagnosed![4]

Even informed doctors can still go wrong when trying to do the right thing. Myths abound about how insurance companies drop people with such preexisting conditions, so patients and some doctors avoid confirming a diagnosis through testing. One such doctor contacted me looking for advice on how to handle a mother and son who were both patients of his and whom he suspected of having celiac disease. He explained to them his perception of the drawbacks of having a firm medical diagnosis in their records and also of having to live gluten-free for the rest of their lives. "You don't know how hard that will be for you, how much it will cost, and how difficult it will be to obtain health insurance," he apparently told them. I impressed upon him about the true costs of ignoring celiac disease and how those far outweighed any initial inconveniences of living gluten-free. Unfortunately, I doubt that this doctor is alone in misunderstanding the true implications of having CD.

Testing for celiac disease is important and should occur in nearly every case in which it is suspected to be at the root of a patient's symptoms. I say *nearly every case* because you should be tested if you or your doctor thinks you might have CD, and you feel that you will not be able to follow a gluten-free diet without a positive diagnosis. Although testing is important for a host of reasons and I advocate it in most cases, I am not one of those who insists that everyone in every circumstance must be tested if he or she suspects the disease. One size does not fit all here; I respect the fact that you

---

4. A. Fasano et al., "A Multi-Center Study on the Sero-Prevalence of Celiac Disease in the United States among Both at Risk and Not at Risk Groups." *Archives of Internal Medicine* 163 (February 2003): 286–92.

Insurance and Celiac Disease

A preexisting condition is a medical condition recognized and present before you enroll in any new group health-care plan. A federal law called **HIPAA** (Health Insurance Portability and Accountability Act of 1996) limits insurance exclusions for **preexisting conditions.** The only preexisting health conditions that may be excluded by a new insurer are those conditions "for which medical advice, diagnosis, care or treatment was recommended or received within the six month period before your enrollment date," or the first day of coverage under the new plan.[5] Therefore, if you had continuous, creditable medical coverage for at least six months without a significant break (over sixty-three days) in coverage prior to your new enrollment, that coverage will offset any preexisting condition exclusion period. Check with your state insurance commissioner's office for details of whether any of these federal HIPAA provisions are extended in your state.

It follows that even if you had a medically diagnosed condition such as celiac disease in the past, but have not received a diagnosis, medical advice, care, or treatment for that condition in the previous six months before enrollment in a new plan, exclusions cannot be applied to this old condition. In general, if you are covered by health insurance when a diagnosis is made, and you maintain health insurance with any carrier thereafter with no break in coverage over sixty-three days, you should be eligible for coverage. Additionally, if you have a job that offers health insurance to its employees, it is typically a group plan that does not exclude individual members due to preexisting conditions. HIPAA also guarantees eligible individuals access to individual policies.

As with any federal or state law, however, it is imperative that you check with an expert in the area to explain how these laws will apply to your particular situation. I recommend that you go first to your state insurance commissioner's office to get answers to your concerns about insurance as it applies to you.

---

5. U.S. Department of Labor, Employee Benefits Security Administration, "Frequently Asked Questions about Portability of Health Coverage and HIPAA," http://www.dol.gov/ebsa/faqs/faq_consumer_hipaa.html.

continues

Another consideration regarding health insurance: if you have a confirmed diagnosis of CD, your health insurance provider should authorize other tests, such as bone density screenings, thyroid tests, and the like. If, prediagnosis, you suffered from related effects of celiac such as depression, having a medical diagnosis of CD may actually help you avoid being excluded or priced out of life or health insurance for those high-risk diagnoses, as well. Furthermore, if medications for celiac disease are approved at any point in the future, it is reasonable to expect insurance companies will not reimburse for those prescriptions unless their insureds have a confirmed diagnosis of CD.

may have unique and valid reasons for not getting tested, so long as you take seriously the need for a lifelong adherence to a gluten-free diet, even if CD is only suspected but not confirmed because testing is not undertaken.

After reading the previous chapter, you should have some idea of how the disease can manifest itself and be disguised by other symptoms. If you now believe that you might have the disease, and you fully appreciate the implications of ignoring the illness, discuss with your physician whether you should be tested. It may be that for you, an official diagnosis is not necessary, since you will be committed to a permanent avoidance of gluten regardless of the diagnosis and you want to be on the road to better health right now! For most, though, a confirmed diagnosis of CD will ensure a lifelong commitment to the diet and reduce the temptation to cheat or even go back to eating gluten regularly, since the genetic implications for relatives of a diagnosed celiac are difficult to ignore. A positive diagnosis of CD within a family may also encourage others to get tested and to become healthy on a gluten-free diet as well.

Furthermore, having baseline bloodwork or biopsy results to use as a comparison at your annual checkup will help to gauge whether you have been successful in your gluten-free diet. If your tests become positive again after first having been negative, it suggests to your doctor that you have perhaps been inadvertently ingesting gluten-containing products. This information could be used to guide you to a specialized nutritionist or other expert in gluten-free living to analyze where contamination has occurred, to help you avoid gluten altogether. Attempting a gluten-free diet is difficult enough, but it would be the worst scenario altogether if you are unwittingly being exposed to gluten and are therefore still sick. (An argument could be made at that point that you might as well be ordering out for pizza if you are going to feel sick anyway!)

For all these reasons, physicians who understand celiac disease will always want their patients whom they suspect of CD to be tested to confirm a diagnosis. This practice is especially important in children. Parents who put their children on a gluten-free diet without testing the youngsters first are making a decision on behalf of their children to adopt a lifestyle change for the rest of their lives. We will discuss other lifestyle issues specific to children in Month 8, but please give thoughtful consideration to the plan of action you undertake for their sake, and maintain regular appointments with a gastroenterologist to help keep you both on track.

IN A SENTENCE

The tests are routine, relatively painless, accurate, and covered by most insurance companies, so in almost every instance they should be undertaken, since celiac patients who fail to adhere to a strict gluten-free diet risk many adverse health consequences.

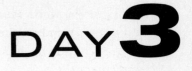

DAY **3**

"What Exactly Is Gluten and Why Doesn't It Like Me?"

GLUTEN IS a food protein found in wheat, barley, and rye. A component of gluten is a substance called gliadin—it is the gliadin found in wheat, barley, and rye gluten that causes the problems for celiacs. Unfortunately, gluten is also the protein that gives many foods and baked goods their signature texture. It lends batters and doughs a taffylike elasticity when they are kneaded or mixed. Gluten also traps the gases formed by fermenting yeast and reacting chemical leavening agents such as baking soda and baking powder, thereby enabling foods like breads to rise. Bake without gluten, and you are likely to find that your cakes, muffins, pastries, and breads will fall apart; and if they rise, they will then fall.

Other grains contain gluten, but they lack the gliadin component that triggers the autoimmune reaction in celiacs and causes the gluten intolerant such digestive difficulties. Corn, for example, contains gluten but is safe for celiacs. However, corn gluten does not perform in the ways that supply the required elasticity for baking. Thus, we must look to other substances in combination with gluten-free grains to provide the binding power necessary for successful baking.

Most grains available today are actually gluten-free. However, wheat is obviously the most prevalent grain in Western societies and it is spreading worldwide (it is second only to corn) as the world economy becomes more intertwined. Interestingly, of all the so-called grass families of grains we find today, only the family associated with wheat, barley, and rye—the Poaceae grass family—is not tolerated by celiacs. Other cereal grains such as oats, rice, and wild rice, as well as pseudocereal grains such as quinoa, flax, amaranth, and the like, are all gluten-free and have been around for millions of years. (Go to my Web site to view a diagram of these grass families. http://NearlyNormalCooking.com/FY/)

Wheat and most other gluten-containing grains are enriched products loaded with important vitamins and minerals. Although many gluten-free grains are full of fiber, protein, and other valuable nutrients, unfortunately many of the most prolific are not. Therefore, switching to an entirely gluten-free diet requires some attention to the nutritional values of replacement grains, to maintain a nutritionally adequate diet. (See Month 10, page 198 for more information on alternative grains.)

It is interesting to note that the grain family containing oats is not on the same line as the wheat branch. Recent studies have proven that, in fact, oats are not problematic for celiacs. However, cross-contamination of oats with other gluten-containing grains in processing facilities remains a source of confusion and concern, thus many celiacs still refrain from eating oats.[1] It makes perfect sense that uncontaminated oats would not cause the same autoimmune reaction if they are from a completely different genus.

A Note on Oats

There has been considerable controversy over whether to exclude oats and oat products from the list of safe, gluten-free grains. It had long been standard protocol to recommend against including oats in a gluten-free diet until more recent studies demonstrated that oats themselves are likely not the source of celiac reaction; rather, the fact that oats are often contaminated with other gluten-containing grains has skewed diagnostic testing of reactions to gluten from oat products. Introducing uncontaminated oats into the celiac diet has many beneficial effects, as oats are an important source of protein and high-

---

1. Recommendations on Oat Consumption, Celiac Center, Beth Israel Deaconess Medical Center (December 2005).

fiber carbohydrates. Furthermore, permitting a wider choice of gluten-free foods will go far toward increasing compliance with a gluten-free diet.

The most recent scientific statements on the inclusion of oats in a gluten-free diet indicate that most individuals with celiac disease can tolerate uncontaminated oats.[2] However, most health professionals (including the American Dietetic Association) recommend that newly diagnosed patients with celiac disease avoid oats until the disease is well controlled with full resolution of symptoms and a normal tissue transglutaminase level (IgA tTG), and that any introduction of oats into the diet of an individual with celiac disease only be done under the guidance of a physician.[3] For celiacs, the recommended daily intake of pure oats should be limited to approximately ¼ cup dry rolled oats for children and ½ to ¾ cup dry rolled oats for adults.[4]

Basic List of Naturally Gluten-Free Foods

This list of examples is by no means comprehensive; rather, it demonstrates the range of naturally gluten-free foods that are safe for those with celiac disease when prepared without gluten-containing ingredients.

Butter	Honey
Chicken	Lentils
Eggs	Meats
Fish	Milk
Fresh fruit and 100% fruit juices	Nuts
Fresh vegetables and 100% vegetable juices	Seeds
Grits	Shellfish
	Sugar

---

2. J. Adams, "New Study Shows Eating Oats Safe for Patients with Celiac Disease," Celiac.com (May 30, 2007).

3. Recommendations on Oat Consumption, Celiac Center, Beth Israel Deaconess Medical Center (December 2005).

4. Health Canada, "Celiac Disease and the Safety of Oats: Health Canada's Position on the Introduction of Oats to the Diet of Individuals Diagnosed with Celiac Disease (CD)," www.hc-sc.gc.ca/fn-an/securi/allerg/cel-coe/oats_cd-avoine_e.html.

Safe Gluten-Free Grain Products

These products are safe in any form, so long as they are not mixed with other non-gluten-free food products or produced in an environment permitting cross-contamination with non-gluten-free foods.

Amaranth	Lentil flour	Sago
Arrowroot	Millet	Seeds (such as sesame)
Buckwheat (including kasha)	Montina	Sorghum
Bean flour	Nut flours (such	Soy
Corn (maize)	as almond meal)	Tapioca (cassava,
Fava bean flour	Potato starch and	manioc)
Flax and flaxseeds	flour	Teff
Garbanzo bean	Quinoa	Wild rice
(chickpea) flour	Rice	

Unsafe or Non-Gluten-Free Grain Products

These products are *not* considered gluten-free in any form or amount.

Bread or bread products	Emmer	Matzo
containing wheat flour	Farina	Modified food starch
(e.g., bread crumbs,	Farro	made from wheat[5]
coating mixes, or Panko)	Graham flour	Orzo and pastina
Barley	Kamut	Rye
Barley malt	Kashi (a trademarked	Seitan
Bulgur	grain blend, not to	Semolina
Couscous	be confused with	Spelt
Durum	kasha)	Triticale
Einkorn	Malt	Wheat

5. In the United States, "modified food starch" or "starch" refers to starches derived from corn or potatoes. Starches derived from other grains, such as wheat, must be noted on the food label. "Following a Gluten-Free Diet," Beth Israel Deaconess Medical Center (January 2006).

Federal food labeling laws and rules have incorporated this recent research and have not excluded oats from future gluten-free labeling, so long as the manufacturer seeking to dub its oats-containing product "gluten-free" must demonstrate that there is less than 20 parts per million (ppm) of gluten in that product, just as in any other gluten-free product.[6] The greatest hurdle in reintroducing oats to a gluten-free diet now appears to be the severe shortage of mills and processing plants that produce certified gluten-free oats, and the resulting excessive costs of those few products.

In 2007, the FDA proposed a rule entitled "**Food-Labeling**: Gluten-free Labeling of Foods," which would define *gluten-free* in the United States. This standard will allow the term *gluten-free* to be voluntarily used on labels, indicating the food is free of the following: any of the prohibited grains of wheat, barley, rye, or their hybrids; ingredients derived from these prohibited grains and that still contain gluten; and any ingredients that contain more than 20 ppm of gluten per gram of food.[7] The final rule, providing for the implementation of the new rule, will likely be issued in 2009.

Reading Labels

Simply understanding the grain basis of gluten in food products is just the beginning, however. It is important to learn to read food labels routinely, as companies often change their ingredients, suppliers, and manufacturing mechanisms and facilities. Always call the manufacturer if you have any questions about ingredients or possible cross-contamination.

I recall that, after my celiac diagnosis in the 1990s, I had very, very few choices for gluten-free foods. I was living in a rural area, the Internet was not at all what it is today, and *gluten-free* and *celiac* were terms that few in this country had ever heard of. One of my early food staples became Kellogg's Corn Pops cereal. Needless to say, without many other alternatives, I got sick of Corn Pops pretty fast; sugared cereals have never really been my thing anyway. One line of a full-page newspaper article about me in 2007 mentioned

---

6. 72 Fed. Reg. 2798.

7. The proposed rule, 72 Fed. Reg. 2795 (January 23, 2007), is available at www.cfsan .fda.gov/~lrd/fr070123.html. FDA's related document, "Questions and Answers on the Gluten-Free Labeling Proposed Rule" (January 23, 2007) is available at www.cfsan.fda.gov/~dms/ glutqa.html.

the fact that I ate a lot of Corn Pops after I was diagnosed. I received scores of e-mails because of that article, and the majority of them pertained to Corn Pops! Either folks were pointing out to me that Corn Pops cereal is not gluten-free or they were questioning whether they could really indeed eat Corn Pops on a gluten-free diet.

This incident is the perfect example of a food manufacturer's changing the ingredients in a well-known product without fanfare or mention. When I was diagnosed, Kellogg's Corn Pops was a gluten-free food; however, at some point in the last few years, Kellogg's quietly changed their recipe for Corn Pops and it is now no longer gluten-free. With a watchful eye, consumers of gluten-free foods have to be fastidious about reading food labels—even of products that they have known to be gluten-free.

Recent changes in the food labeling laws in the United States have thankfully made the job of reading and understanding food labels much easier for celiacs, gluten intolerant, and wheat allergic people alike.[8] The Food Allergen Labeling and Consumer Protection Act (**FALCPA**) of 2004 requires that manufacturers must list on a product label any of the eight main food allergens (milk, egg, peanuts, tree nuts, fish, shellfish, soy, and wheat) if they are contained in that manufactured product or if they are secondary ingredients to the spices, natural or artificial flavorings, additives, or colorings.[9] The law covers food products, dietary supplements, and vitamins, but it does not apply to over-the-counter medications or to prescription drugs (see Month 7 for more information on these items).

FALCPA requires the Food and Drug Administration (FDA) to issue a final rule to define and permit the voluntary use of the term *gluten-free* on food labels no later than August 2008.[10] The FDA has proposed to define the term

8. Food Allergen Labeling and Consumer Protection Act of 2004 (FALCPA), 21 U.S.C. § 301 et Seq., Public Law 108–282, Title II, available at www.cfsan.fda.gov/~dms/alrgact.html.

9. American Celiac Disease Alliance Food Labeling (FALCPA) Fact Sheet (November 2005), http://americanceliac.org/ACDA%20Food%20Labeling%20Fact%20Sheet%2011–05Final.pdf; Food allergies: Food labels list top 8 allergens; Food labels list the top eight allergens to help you avoid an allergic reaction, MayoClinic.com, www.mayoclinic.com/health/food-allergies/AA00057 (January 3, 2007).

10. Information for Consumers: Food Allergen Labeling And Consumer Protection Act of 2004: Questions and Answers, USFDA Center for Food Safety and Applied Nutrition (July 18, 2006), http://www.cfsan.fda.gov/~dms/alrgqa.html#q11.

gluten-free for voluntary use in the labeling of foods, thereby allowing a manufacturer to label its product gluten-free, free from gluten, without gluten or no gluten if it chooses to do so, and, if the food product bearing this label meets the proposed regulatory definition of no more than 20 ppm per gram of food.[11] As research and laws are constantly changing, and not every country accepts the same standards for what is gluten-free or low gluten, you would be wise to always check label standards from products manufactured and sold outside of the United States.[12] Even within this country, you should be cautious with products purporting to be gluten-free but lacking an adequate ingredient label (such as breads sold at farmers' markets).

Although these food labeling changes are welcomed, they may usher in a host of new problems. As manufacturers attempt to comply with the labeling laws, and as food allergies and intolerances multiply in actual and perceived number, more labels will be filled with cautionary language that the food consumer must sort through. A recent article in *Newsweek* magazine discussed the fact that the food warnings are already so common on labels that consumers are increasingly ignoring them. Caveats such as "may contain" or "made on equipment that also produces" muddy the waters for label readers in their search for truly safe products. Apparently, parents of children with food allergies and intolerances are increasingly ignoring them; a study in 2007 indicated that 75 percent of these parents claimed to pay attention to these type of cautionary labels, down from 85 percent in 2003.[13] Since even more labeling rules will be in place soon, one has to wonder if that statistic will trend down even further in the near future.

---

11. C. Catassi et al., "A Prospective, Double-Blind, Placebo-Controlled Trial to Establish a Safe Gluten Threshold for Patients with Celiac Disease," *American Journal of Clinical Nutrition* 85(2007): 160–66; 21 CFR Part 101, "Food Labeling; Gluten-Free Labeling of Foods" (January 23, 2007).

12. The Codex Alimentarius Commission, created by the World Health Organization and the Food and Agriculture Organization of the United Nations, provides the only international gluten-free food standard for manufacturers. Its members do not include every country, however. The Codex Alimentarius currently specifies that naturally gluten-free products contain less than 20 ppm of gluten, and products that are rendered gluten-free, such as "Codex wheat starch," contain less than 200 ppm of gluten. "Research Study on the Establishment of a Safe Gluten Threshold for Celiac Disease Patients," S. Adams, Celiac.com (January 10, 2007), www.celiac.com/articles/1095/1/Research-Study-on-the-Establishment-of-a-Safe-Gluten-Threshold-for-Celiac-Disease-Patients/Page1.html.

13. Claudia Kalb, "Fear and Allergies in the Lunchroom," *Newsweek* 47 (November 5, 2007).

Other Common Products and Ingredients That MAY Contain Gluten

Baking powder

Bread crumbs

Brown rice syrup

Candy, including some chocolates

Cereals

Chewing gum (may be dusted in gluten-containing flour before being wrapped)

Communion wafers

Croutons

Cured pork products

Dextrin

Drink mixes

Drugs (both prescription and over-the-counter medications)

Flavored coffees and teas

Flavorings or seasonings

Gelatin

Glue and adhesive (such as envelope adhesive)

Hydrolyzed vegetable protein (HVP)

Hydrolyzed plant protein (HPP)

Imitation seafood or bacon

Licorice

Malts and milk shakes

Malt and malt flavorings

Modified starch and modified food starch (in the United States, though, modified food starch is now gluten-free unless otherwise indicated on the label; see footnote 5)

Nutritional supplements and vitamins

Pasta

Play dough (if ingested)

Processed meats

Sauces (soy sauce, gravy, marinades, etc.)

Self-basting poultry

Soups and broths (cans, cartons, and cubes)

Starch

Stuffing and dressing

Texturized Vegetable Protein (TVP)

Thickeners (such as roux)[14]

---

14. See "Reading Ingredient Labels," Food Allergy Initiative, www.foodallergyinitiative.org/images/allergen_free_bro.pdf.

IN A SENTENCE

You'll need to make it your mission to understand gluten, to recognize the grains you can and can't include in your diet, and to learn to read labels effectively and continually.

living

"How Can I Have a Disease I Have Never Heard Of?"

I BELIEVE that most of us share some sense of disbelief upon learning of the possibility that we have a disease. *Disease* carries with it such negative, ominous connotations. In your own journey to diagnosis, you may have been told many different things along the way, and this latest diagnosis of CD probably seems as uncertain as any other. Or perhaps you learned of your illness almost accidentally, and wonder if you can't just go back to being blissfully ignorant of the disease. In my case, I initially doubted the qualifications of the physician who made the diagnosis since I had seen so many seemingly more expert doctors before him who had run every other possible test and determined that I must have had IBS.

I did not want to be told that I had a disease, but perhaps even worse was being told that I could not ever again eat all of the things that I had enjoyed my whole life. Never again?! The implications of this life change were beyond my comprehension. I suddenly realized how big a role food played in my daily life and how suddenly ordinary things seemed much more complicated. How could I go out to eat with my work colleagues?

How could I go on a date? How could I pack a picnic? How could I entertain? How could I eat at a friend's house? How could I participate in Thanksgiving with my family? How could I have a birthday party? Was this disease going to cause my friends to avoid including me in social settings? Was embarrassment for me or for them worth changing my life? How much was this disease going to hurt me if I didn't change the way I ate?

I hear from people every day who share these concerns and who worry over the life change that they must suddenly undertake when diagnosed with CD. Fear of this unknown is justification for some to avoid testing for celiac disease and to pretend that they don't have it, no matter what the costs.

I am convinced that my grandmother had CD (my mother and I both do), yet she wouldn't hear of it. No matter that she had numerous chronic intestinal difficulties, rheumatoid arthritis at middle age, fibromyalgia, early heart disease, degenerative joints and back pain, headaches, and who knows what else she wouldn't tell us about. The fear of having to change her diet, of not being able to participate in church socials or eat with her family at reunions and holidays, was enough to convince her not to even mention the possibility to her doctors. She died a painful death at the age of seventy-two and now my grandmother is gone. I miss her terribly and wish that there was some way to turn back time and inspire a physician along the way to insist that she be tested; she would have listened to a doctor tell her she needed a test. If I had been able to show her then what I know now—that gluten-free life without pain is such a gift—I wonder if my grandmother would still be with us.

It Could Be Worse

You could do a lot worse than earn yourself a diagnosis of celiac disease. It may not feel like that on day three, but you will soon come to understand that this diagnosis is more of a blessing than it is a curse. You will certainly ride waves of self-pity, guilt, and confusion about having this disease, but those waves will decrease in number and severity over time until you realize that you have essentially been given a gift of control over your health destiny.

How much attention have you ever really paid before to what you put into your body? Did you know whether you were getting the appropriate nutritional value out of your food, or were you simply eating whatever was around because it tasted good or was convenient, quick, and easy? If someone told you that you could go a long way toward preventing myriad future diseases and extending your life by simply revising your diet, wouldn't you feel fortunate to be given the choice? Whether or not you were severely sick before your diagnosis, isn't it nice to know that on a gluten-free diet, you probably won't be severely sick in the future? What other conditions can be prevented without taking medications? Whenever I doubt the benefits of my diagnosis, I remind myself of these arguments and I truly feel much better about my health and my future.

Depending on how sick you were at the time of your own diagnosis (or when you suspect you might have CD), you might be tempted to ignore the signs, disbelieve the science, and just "deal with the symptoms," as one of my consulting clients put it. Cheating by eating gluten in moderation or on occasion is another route some people choose to take. However, it is irresponsible of any physician who grasps the severity of the disease to counsel against testing or against adherence to a gluten-free diet for those who are diagnosed. CD is not simply about symptoms and inconvenient eating habits. It is not an allergy nor is it a simple intolerance; it is a serious autoimmune disease that, if ignored, can and will lead to other serious health issues.[15] To refuse testing or refuse to accept a diagnosis is akin to allowing your body to be damaged from the inside out.

Adjusting to life with CD is a dramatic life change, but it is one in which you have the opportunity to embrace your life, protect your health, and change your future simply by putting different things on your table and into your mouth. Once I realized the severity of the disease I have and once I learned how to make all of my favorite foods again safely, I had no reason to ever look back, and neither will you.

IN A SENTENCE

> *Celiac disease is not something to be ignored, and a gluten-free diet is not something to "sort of" follow—but once you realize that you now have control over your future health, you will gradually come to accept and even to embrace a diagnosis of an exclusively diet-controlled disease.*

---

15. See www.americanceliac.org, the Web site of the American Celiac Disease Alliance.

learning

Everything You Never Wanted to Know about Your Intestines (and Were Hoping You Wouldn't Need to Ask!)

TO UNDERSTAND how celiac disease affects your body, you must begin with a basic understanding of your intestines. Your gastrointestinal tract is divided into two sections: the small, or upper intestine and the large, or lower intestine. The small intestine joins the stomach to the large intestine and is where most of the body's digestion occurs, absorbing virtually all food nutrients into the blood. The large intestine is the final portion of the digestive system; it absorbs any remaining water from indigestible food and flushes the leftovers from the body.

If you could see your small intestines as physicians do during upper endoscopic procedures, they should look like they are lined with thick 1970s shag carpeting. The shag carpet is comprised of villi, which are vital to the body's absorption of fluids, minerals, vitamins, and other key nutrients from food. Furthermore, the surface of the villi themselves produce enzymes, such as lactase, which break down food particles (in this example, milk sugar, or lactose), enabling proper digestion.

In a person with active celiac disease, the spaces between cells lining the small intestine open too widely or get stuck open and allow large gluten molecules to absorb into the upper intestine. These absorbed proteins, such as gluten and other allergens, then stimulate the body's immune system, triggering an immune response that causes chronic inflammation and damages the villi. Once this is set into motion, various sections of villi become blunted or even completely flattened (to complete the analogy, they become matted like industrial-grade Berber carpeting), effectively preventing the efficient absorption of food and leading to the symptoms of celiac disease.[1]

Obvious problems may result, such as malnutrition, weight loss, diarrhea, gas and bloating, and reduced bone density. Over time, other organ systems are dragged down as well.

An important distinction between the effects of celiac disease and those caused by a food allergy is that the physical reaction to the allergen is directly linked to eating that particular allergen, whereas the intestinal damage caused by celiac disease lingers no matter what is for dinner. To put it another way, a person with a food allergy usually experiences a negative physical reaction upon exposure to a particular food allergen. A person with active CD will have the same physical problems (bloating, gas, diarrhea, constipation, malabsorption, and so on) whether he or she eats a gluten-free salad or a Big Mac. Operating with damaged villi, a body cannot properly digest anything, not just gluten. The ingestion of gluten causes the damage to a celiac body and causes the damage to persist and to worsen but does not need to occur with every meal for that celiac to feel negative effects.

Don't Cheat!

Individuals recover from gluten damage at different rates, just as they exhibit differing symptoms because of that damage. Improvements in health typically begin within days of starting a strict gluten-free diet, although it can take up to three to six months for younger people and two years for older

---

1. Researchers Find Increased Zonulin Levels among Celiac Disease Patients, May 1, 2000, http://www.umm.edu/news/releases/zonulin.htm.

adults to have completely healed intestinal villi.[2] It is evident, then, that the length of time between your last gluten-filled lunch and your next gluten-free meal that does not make you feel sick can vary widely. All of these problems not only contribute to the difficulty of diagnosing CD but also to the temptation to think that going gluten-free might not be working for you since it does not necessarily make you feel better right away. This delay is often why people cheat. No matter how long it takes for you to return to a symptom-free life though, it is crucial to give your body the time to heal through a gluten-free diet and to maintain that diet for the rest of your life.

Research has shown that *any* amount of gluten can damage the intestinal villi of a person with celiac disease (even as little as $1/8$ teaspoon of gluten—approximately 1/1000, or .05 percent of a slice of bread). Even without symptoms, you are still risking medical complications from celiac disease if you do not follow a strict gluten-free diet and avoid cross-contamination (see page 7).[3] As of now, there are no alternatives to living gluten-free for those of us with CD. Given the volume and variety of wonderful foods you can safely consume without causing harm, there is really no reason to "cheat" and endanger your future health.

New Advances

Despite the fact that a gluten-free diet will always be crucial to celiacs, significant recent advances toward further understanding the physiology of celiac disease have made the possibility of finding pharmaceutical remedies or preventative measures to CD a reality. The University of Maryland's innovative Center for Celiac Research, in particular, has made great strides in this arena, discovering an intestinal protein called "**zonulin**" that regulates intestinal permeability (it acts as a gatekeeper, opening and closing doors in the gastrointestinal tract to allow nutrients to pass through and prevent bacteria and other toxins from slipping through).[4] Gluten exposure in people with celiac disease

---

2. Healthlink, "Celiac Disease," Medical College of Wisconsin, http://healthlink.mcw.edu/article/956622658.html.

3. Ibid.

4. M. G. Clemente et al., "Early Effects of Gliadin on Enterocyte Intracellular Signalling Involved in Intestinal Barrier Function," *Gut* 52, no. 2 (February 2003): 218–23; A. Fasano et al., "Zonulin, a Newly Discovered Modulator of Intestinal Permeability, and Its Expression in Cœliac Disease," *Lancet* 355 (2000): 1518–19.

causes an increase in zonulin production, thereby increasing their intestinal permeability to the point of actual leakage between the intestines and other body compartments. These intercellular spaces, or tight junctions, which open too widely in people with celiac disease, allow large molecules of gluten proteins to slip through and trigger damaging autoimmune inflammation.

A new drug called AT–1001 is proving in clinical trials that it may be possible to reduce the permeability of these tight junctions, preventing gluten proteins from ever entering the intestinal lining, and removing the impetus for any autoimmune (celiac) response.[5] Other approaches, such as oral enzyme therapy, might actually counter the toxic celiac effects from small amounts of food containing gluten. Clinical trials for drugs like these raise the hopes of a treatment for celiac as well as other autoimmune diseases in the not so distant future.[6]

IN A SENTENCE

> *Understanding your body's gastrointestinal system and the internal effects of celiac disease can help you embrace the importance of a gluten-free diet; although we may one day be able to look forward to a drug, for now we will still have to rely on a gluten-free diet.*

---

5. "Alba Therapeutics Announces Phase IIb Clinical Trial for Oral AT–1001 for the Treatment of Celiac Disease," Baltimore, Md., September 19, 2007, PRNewswire.

6. S. Galante, "Beyond Gluten-Free: Two Companies Are Making Progress on Non-Dietary Treatments for Celiac," CeliacToday.com (December 2007); M. Ludvig and K. Chaitan, "Future Therapeutic Options for Celiac Disease," *Nature Clinical Practice Gastroenterology Hepatology* 2, no. 3 (2005): 140–47; J. Adams, "A Sweet Pill for Celiacs to Swallow? Progress on Enzyme Therapy for Celiac Disease," Celiac.com (February 7, 2008).

living

"You're in Control": Susie Delaney's Story

THAT YOUR condition can be controlled through diet alone is quite a blessing. Susie Delaney suffered so many painful symptoms before being correctly diagnosed with celiac disease that she was grateful for any relief, no matter what form. She soon realized that relief for celiacs comes in the form of something that does not require a prescription pad or rigorous medical treatments. Her newfound health and healthy outlook on a gluten-free life are inspirational to us all.

◇ ◇ ◇

Susie Delaney's Story

Congratulations! You are lucky enough to be diagnosed with the only known disease that grants the patient total control. Feeling good, having energy, and leading a normal life again is only a choice away. You are about to reclaim your spirit, be introduced to an exciting new world of food, and change your life in ways you can't possibly imagine. From this point on, being healthy is simply a choice.

I am grateful to be part of this growing club of celiacs and I hope after reading my story, you will be, too.

By the time I was diagnosed, celiac disease had claimed every cell in my body. I was completely debilitated. Over the years, I never lost hope that I would find a diagnosis, but my spirit was sufficiently broken. I was fearful that doctors, nurses, needles, hospitals, health insurance, prescription drugs, and lab tests would dominate the better part of my years. My journey to diagnosis was scary, defeating, and terribly lonely. By the end, I had trouble sleeping, partially because of physical discomfort and partially because my most intimate fears would emerge in the silence of the night. Would I ever feel like myself again? Was making it to the end of the day in one piece always going to be this difficult? Who would fall in love with a twenty-four-year-old with so many health problems? How would I afford my inevitable medical plight? And on and on. It was too much stress for a young woman.

I needed something positive to hold onto. Just when I thought I couldn't bear another misleading diagnosis or invasive medical test, hope came in the form of celiac disease. During a routine visit, my primary care physician told me I was lactose intolerant and I might have celiac. I had never heard of it. I was told to lay off dairy and come back in six weeks; if I didn't feel better, he'd test me for CD. I went home and Googled *celiac disease*. I had every symptom. I called my mother and told her to look it up. It took her a minute to respond. When she finally spoke, I realized she was crying. She said, "Susie, call that doctor back and tell him you need to be tested today." I did . . . and I was! (See list of possible symptoms, pages 6–7.) The *only* symptom I didn't have was weight loss! I mean really, what does a girl have to do to drop a few pounds?!

That same day I went back to the hospital and had blood drawn. I started the diet the next day. Five days later, I woke up a new person: no headache, no joint pain, no cramping. I was beginning to heal. That was the beginning of a new life. Celiac disease changed me in ways I never thought possible. At a very young age, it forced me to decide what was most important in my life. It empowered me to take responsibility for my health and happiness. And it allowed me to become a more grateful, joyous, loving person. I would not trade a piece of pizza, a beer, an English muffin, or a hamburger bun for the way I feel when I wake up in the morning. I certainly wouldn't trade my diagnosis for one that requires medication, excessive blood tests, scans, and hospital visits. Everyone has his or her cross to bear and I couldn't be happier that this is mine.

Every time someone I love sends me an article, researches and prepares a gluten-free menu, chooses a restaurant with my diet in mind, questions a waiter on my behalf, or places a special order and then travels across town to bring me gluten-free cupcakes on my birthday, it is an overt sign of that person's love for me. What an amazing gift. I have a disease where the cure lies within me and the treatment is something that everyone around me can participate in.

Now that you're part of the club, you should ask yourself one question, "How far am I willing to go to take care of myself and reclaim my health?" Be honest. Don't be resentful—that's negative energy, and negative energy is a waste of your time. Be grateful. I guarantee any cancer patient on the planet would trade places with you. Can you imagine if curing cancer was as simple as removing gluten from your diet? Wow.

It took a little practice, but I'm now a fully functioning celiac. I eat at wonderful restaurants, sometimes up to four or five times a week! I go to client lunches, I entertain friends, I tailgate, I go to parties, and I travel both domestically and internationally. I've learned to do it all with a positive outlook and relative ease, and so will you. If you let it, celiac disease will introduce you to the most amazing parts of yourself and bring you a level of satisfaction that you've never before experienced.

If you want to be a grateful celiac, here are my two cents . . . mope around for a couple days, stuff your face with one last pepperoni pizza, wash it down with a beer, and *move on*! You've been sick for too long to waste time mourning food. Trust me, I'm not sitting at home wondering where my next meal will come from—I eat everything I can. There's a whole world of wonderful alternative grains and savory gluten-free food combinations just waiting to be discovered. Don't explore that world alone. Be excited about your newfound health and others will, too.

Congratulations! You're entering an exciting, new world where your health and happiness are within your control. Take the tools that are in this book and start living; expect more for yourself and for the people you love. You'll be amazed at the possibilities gluten-free living holds!

◇ ◇ ◇

IN A SENTENCE

> *Embrace the fact that your condition can be managed through diet alone, and adopt a positive outlook on your new future in which you are in control of your own health and happiness.*

learning

The History of Celiac Disease (and Its Current Statistical Prevalence)

CELIAC DISEASE was not always recognized as being linked to diet. It was actually first identified in second century Greece simply as a malabsorptive syndrome causing chronic diarrhea. It was termed a "cœliac affection," coming from the Greek word *koiliakos* for abdominal region.[1] In the 1800s, some connection was made between these symptoms and improper digestion, but it was not until the late 1880s that a pediatrician in London described the condition as one affecting children and adults that could only be "cured" through diet. At that time, although starches were recognized as problematic for these sufferers, rice, fruit, and vegetables were incorrectly restricted in favor of raw meat and thin slices of toast! In 1924, American pediatrician Sydney V. Haas reported success in celiacs, by means of a diet exclusively comprised of bananas. This extremely restrictive diet was prescribed until the link was finally made between CD and wheat in 1950.

---

1. Wikipedia, "Coeliac Disease," http://en.wikipedia.org/wiki/Coeliac_disease.

World War II—and specifically the Dutch famine of 1944—provided the first large-scale opportunity to observe a link between elimination of wheat flour in the diet and the amelioration of clinical symptoms of celiac disease. Dutch pediatrician W. K. Dicke noticed that the incidence of celiac disease was reduced during wartime grain scarcities in Holland. When the war ended and wheat and other grains returned to the table, the clinical improvement in celiac symptoms, which had occurred so markedly during the wartime shortages, surprisingly disappeared with the peacetime resumption of grain availability. Soon thereafter, a link was made with the gluten component of wheat. Villous atrophy was finally identified in 1954, once intestinal biopsies obtained during abdominal surgeries were available.[2]

Until quite recently, no other major discoveries about celiac disease had been made, largely because it was thought that the disease was quite rare. Conventional wisdom in the United States held that only 1 in 10,000 Americans had the disease. In 2003, however, Dr. Alessio Fasano of the University of Maryland's Center for Celiac Research published the results of one of the largest epidemiological studies ever performed in the United States. The multicenter study was undertaken between February 1996 and May 2001 and included over thirteen thousand subjects comprised of an age distribution that closely corresponded to the population of the 2000 census and resided in thirty-two states. This remarkable study demonstrated that celiac disease actually affects 1 in 133 Americans, or approximately 3 million people—a prevalence rate similar to that reported in Europe—making it one of the most frequent chronic genetic disorders of humankind.[3]

Not surprisingly, these statistics are similar to those demonstrating the prevalence of celiac disease in Europeans and also show that CD can affect any ethnic background, not just Caucasians as originally thought. Universal acceptance of this study has put celiac disease on the research radar, but the disease still remains vastly underdiagnosed by physicians, since as much as 97 percent of those with CD are as yet undiagnosed.[4]

---

2. Wikipedia, "Coeliac Disease," http://en.wikipedia.org/wiki/Coeliac_disease.

3. A. Fasano et al., "A Multi-Center Study on the Sero-Prevalence of Celiac Disease in the United States among Both at Risk and Not at Risk Groups," *Archives of Internal Medicine* 163 (February 2003): 286–92.

4. A. Fasano et al., "A Multi-Center Study."

How Does Prevalence
of Celiac Disease Compare?[5]

Illness	Number of American Sufferers
Celiac Disease	at least 3 million Americans
Autism	556,000 Americans
Crohn's disease	500,000 Americans
Cystic fibrosis	30,000 Americans
Down syndrome	350,000 Americans (42,000 of those diagnosed also have celiac disease)
Epilepsy	2.7 million Americans
Hemophilia	17,000 Americans
Infertility (unexplained)	610,000 American women (36,600 of those also have celiac disease)
Lupus	1.5 million Americans
Multiple sclerosis	400,000 Americans
Parkinson's disease	1 million Americans
Rheumatoid arthritis	2.1 million Americans
Type 1 diabetes	3 million Americans (180,000 of those diagnosed also have celiac disease)
Ulcerative colitis	500,000 Americans

5. University of Chicago Celiac Disease Program, "Celiac Disease Fact Sheet," http://www.uchospitals.edu/pdf/uch_007937.pdf.

Despite recent statistical evidence effectively demonstrating that celiac disease affects millions, the vast majority of those sufferers remain undiagnosed. Statistics are not uniformly available for every country; even so, studies are beginning to show that celiac is common not just among northern European populations, and also that it may be more common than previously thought even in Africa, South America, and Asia.[6] Celiac disease is only just starting to receive the medical and research attention its prevalence deserves.

IN A SENTENCE

> *Although celiac disease was recognized for centuries as a wasting condition in children and later in adults, only within the latter part of the twentieth century was it linked to eating certain cereal grains and, in the last five years, have researchers begun to appreciate that it affects tens of millions of people worldwide.*

6. "Celiac Disease," National Digestive Diseases Information Clearinghouse (NDDIC), http://digestive.niddk.nih.gov/ddiseases/pubs/celiac/index.htm#7.

living

My, How Times Have Changed!
Barbara Hudson's Story

WHATEVER DIFFICULTIES you may experience because of your diagnosis with celiac disease, we should all be grateful that medical advances have pinpointed gluten exposure as the trigger for CD. Those treated as recently as the twentieth century suffered under exceedingly restrictive diets that give us true perspective into the relatively minor restrictions we now have. Barbara Hudson shares her unique experience of having been treated for celiac disease in the early 1900s and being treated again under the new guidelines established in this century.

◇ ◇ ◇

Barbara Hudson's Story

At birth on February 14, 1936, I weighed 8 pounds 2 ounces. According to my mother, I was a healthy baby until I got the measles in April 1937. At that time I started having problems. They had nothing to do with measles, of course, but started because I was then eating table foods. In my baby book there is a statement that I *was not thriving*.

Our family doctor told my parents to take me to a pediatrician in Baltimore. That was quite a trip then, as there were no interstate highways, and it took over an hour each way from our family farm north of the city. On July 4, 1937, I was taken for ten days to what was then University Hospital but did not improve. Then on September 21, 1937, my mother dropped me off at the hospital a second time and was told to not come to see me for six weeks. I ended up staying in the hospital until June 28, 1938—nine months and one week. One of my first memories is that of standing in a crib and looking through a window at nurses sitting at a desk on the other side.

Dr. Loring Joslin was my pediatrician and diagnosed my problem as celiac disease. We don't know how he did that at that time, but my diet became what we knew as baked bananas and Bulgarian buttermilk (the "**Banana Diet**"), which I now think contained dehydrated banana powder. There was another little boy in the hospital with me with the same problems. We were documented in a 1938 university medical journal as being *first survivors*. In Dr. Joslin's obituary in 1958, he was credited as being the first physician to show the value of pectin and dehydrated banana powder in the treatment of diarrhea in infants and children.

I lived on the baked bananas and Bulgarian buttermilk for two or three years, and in all that time, my mother never tasted it, as it looked so terrible. Bananas were not easy to buy back then, either. A family member or a friend had to go to Baltimore each week to purchase the twenty-one-banana weekly supply (three bananas a day for seven days a week).

My mother was told I would outgrow the condition, so other foods were gradually added to my diet and seemed to be tolerated. Dairy products were the last to be added, so by age six, I was allowed to eat ice cream.

During elementary school and high school I had diarrhea many times, but no doctor connected it to celiac disease. In spite of that, I thought I was cured. After college I married, taught kindergarten, and had four sons. I had no problems during any of the pregnancies. In 1963, I was diagnosed with dermatitis herpetiformis (DH) at the University of Michigan Hospital in Ann Arbor, Michigan. Drugs, not diet, were used to control it. Again, no connection was made back to celiac disease.

As an adult, my diarrhea returned occasionally, and in 1968 it lasted two months. I did not feel it was life threatening, just an inconvenience. I could never be farther away from a bathroom than ten minutes' time, if that. My sister did all my Christmas shopping for me that year, as I could not be away from the house long enough. Doctors again did not connect this to celiac disease. In fact, it was ascribed to nerves.

In 1984, we were living in Connecticut and after a physical I was told that I was very anemic, which I had been all my life, and that I had a blood count of 7, when 12 to 14 is normal. The doctor said my blood cells also "looked funny." I was sent to a gastroenterologist, and again I told him my medical history. He told me that I could not have celiac disease because the test was not invented until the 1970s. He did a biopsy and, sure enough, it showed that I had celiac disease, as the villi in my small intestine were flat. I never went back to that doctor again. I also had a skin biopsy right after that, and it showed the DH.

Since that time, I have eaten a gluten-free diet. My skin cleared up and my GI tract is in much better shape. My sister also has celiac disease. She was diagnosed in 1976 at Union Memorial Hospital in Baltimore. At the time my mother was relieved to learn my sister only had celiac disease and not cancer. It was not easy for either of us to find gluten-free food products and recipes back then. Even though she was in Maryland and I was in Connecticut, when we found something new, we would share ideas and foods.

There were no support groups where I lived at that time, but I became one myself by reputation. I found I was able to help other people. One night, a woman came to my house in tears. Her eight-year-old daughter had just been diagnosed with celiac disease. The daughter was upset because she could never eat Oreo cookies again. I told her that was correct but also told her of a lot of things she could eat and that there are many other diseases that are a lot worse. The woman left with a new confidence.

Today, it is much easier to find gluten-free products, even in our local grocery stores. I still do a lot of cooking myself, especially soups. (At this writing, there are six or seven different kinds in the freezer for the winter.) I try to carry something with me that I can eat if I am going to be out at mealtime, particularly when traveling. On the other hand, when we have taken major trips, proper food has always been available.

I know that people with celiac disease can live a good life. I am healthier than are many of my friends of the same age. This disease may have been a battle at times, but on the whole, my life has been very good. My husband of almost fifty years, my four sons, and my twelve grandchildren can attest to that. So here I am, your banana baby.

IN A SENTENCE

> *We should count our blessings that modern research has identified gluten exposure as the trigger for celiac disease, since the elimination of gluten from our diets is far easier to live with than earlier treatments prescribing total elimination of all food sources except bananas.*

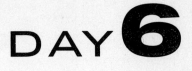

learning

"Why Me? Why Now?"

AT THIS point you may be asking yourself, "How did I get celiac disease? Could I have done something to prevent this?"

We still do not know why celiac disease manifests itself so differently in different people, and why the symptoms develop early in some and very much later in others. Many factors are currently under study that can help us learn whether we can thwart or delay the onset by introducing gluten-containing foods to children earlier, by delaying its introduction for a period of time, by reducing the amount of gluten exposure, or even by breast-feeding for a longer period of time. We can look forward to having the benefit of these and other studies specifically aimed at celiac disease in the not-so-distant future.

These academic questions are important for society at large, but the most crucial point for you to accept and understand is that *you have done nothing wrong*. If you have been diagnosed with celiac disease, it is only because you were genetically predisposed to have it. If you lacked certain genes—at this time researchers have identified the presence of HLA-DQ2 and HLA-DQ8 as the most accurate markers of genetic predisposition for CD—then no amount of eating gluten would give you celiac disease.[1] You may have an intolerance for gluten or a wheat allergy (due to other environmental and perhaps genetic factors), but you would not have celiac disease.

Certain risk factors can contribute to the onset of symptoms if you are genetically predisposed to CD. Again, these risk factors are not your fault. Pregnancy, age at puberty onset, injury or trauma, surgeries, infections (viral or bacterial), other autoimmune diseases, antibiotic or other medication use causing alterations in the flora or other injury to the gut, or any other stress may initiate the celiac reaction in an already predisposed individual. Once that chain reaction is begun, it is lifelong and currently irreversible. Interestingly, recent studies have confirmed that a correlation need not exist between the extent of actual intestinal damage and overt symptoms in celiac patients. Celiac disease may become active, but the individual may not realize any symptoms that would lead him or her to seek medical attention for any number of years. This delay contributes to the difficulty in diagnosing CD and to the differing amounts of intestinal damage present upon each person's final diagnosis.[2]

So, once you relieve yourself of any burden of guilt from contracting this disease, you can move on to a healthier place: to deal with and benefit from the knowledge that you can control your symptoms and minimize your chances of future disease and illness by simply avoiding gluten and taking charge of your health. Since you did not do anything to cause yourself to get this disease, there is no point in looking back—only forward to a healthier, happier life where your deliberate actions can alleviate your painful and uncomfortable symptoms!

One other thing you will want to consider and discuss with your physician is whether, as a result of undiagnosed celiac disease or from other causes, you have any existing nutrient deficiencies. If so, your physician or nutritionist will probably encourage you to take some nutritional supplements in addition to a high-quality multivitamin. Some of the kinds of nutrients you may want to supplement are vitamins B_{12}, B_6, K, and E. Folic acid and calcium

1. National Institutes of Health Consensus Development Conference Final Statement: Celiac Disease (August 9, 2004).

2. Mayo Clinic, "Mayo Clinic Finds Capsule Endoscopy Can Detect Intestinal Damage Caused by Celiac Disease: Study Shows Extent of Intestinal Damage Does Not Explain Patients' Symptoms," http://www.mayoclinic.org/news2008-rst/4669.html (February 27, 2008).

are two additional supplements that many celiacs should consider adding to their vitamin regimen. Depending on your symptoms, you may also find that probiotics are beneficial for you. Make sure you check with your pharmacist if you are at all unclear from the labels of any of these products whether they are gluten-free, and always ask your doctor's advice on any supplementation.

IN A SENTENCE

Genetic predisposition and certain risk factors can contribute to the onset of symptoms of celiac disease, but it is crucial to remember that you didn't do anything wrong to make this happen.

living

The Essential Ingredient to Living Gluten-Free

WE'VE ESTABLISHED that you should not feel guilty about having CD, so now you must be convinced not to feel overwhelmed by it! You may have already met with a physician or even a dietitian who has left you feeling pessimistic about your lifestyle from now on. I urge you to set aside any of those negative, fearful emotions, however difficult that might be. You must move forward and make a new, better, healthier life for yourself, and so you shall. It is possible and you are not alone.

Start with a plan of action. In the next few days, you will clear out your kitchen and you will go shopping. Before we undertake that, though, I want to introduce you to the essential ingredient that will carry you through the rest of your gluten-free life and will return the sense of optimism to you that much of the medical and dietetic community have unwittingly removed due to their lack of intimacy with a gluten-free diet.

So many dishes and baked goods include enriched white flour or wheat flour—which people who have celiac cannot tolerate. The often overlooked yet essential ingredient to a successful gluten-free diet is a really good, *all-purpose* gluten-free flour. By really good, I mean one that you can substitute one-for-one for wheat-based flours in all your recipes without sacrificing their flavor. Translation: this essential ingredient will allow you to make all your favorite recipes again, and eat them safely.

We will get into the intricacies of all the potential gluten-free flours you could use to develop such a mix (and the food science properties of such a mix) in the final chapter of this book. For now, though, imagine that I am with you at your kitchen table and am passing to you my tattered recipe card for the base of my favorite recipes. I will give you the recipe that gave me my life back. You can use it to speed your own recovery to a "normal" life with celiac disease.

Years of experimentation and inventing the gluten-free wheel, back when no really good recipes or mixes were available, taught me everything I know about gluten-free flours and recipes. But none of the details of those facts made half of the difference in my daily life that this flour mixture has. It is not just that this mixture is wonderful, doesn't taste gritty, is not dry or crumbly, and doesn't leave an aftertaste (all hallmarks of most gluten-free food), it is the very fact that I can now have a single flour sitting on my shelf like every other person (without celiac) does in their kitchens. When I want to make a recipe, I simply add the required measurement of my flour mix to the recipe and move on to the other ingredients, just like every other cook. With a supply of this flour on hand, I don't have to worry about adding additional binders to a mixture. I no longer concern myself with starch-to-flour ratios. Nor do I have to stop midrecipe to pull six different flours off the shelf to make a recipe my neighbor would have made with one scoop from her Gold Medal flour bag.

I hear some folks say that you need to use different gluten-free flours in each type of recipe to achieve optimum results. But most of us don't have the luxury of extra time, energy, shelf space, and money to spend on all these different types of gluten-free flour every time we make a new recipe. I devised my own all-purpose gluten-free flour mixture and I use it in every kind of recipe—from apple crisp to cupcakes, pizza, roux, zucchini bread, and everything in between—and I could hardly ask for a better result! Why make life any harder than it has to be?

So, whether you use my all-purpose mixture, devise your own, or purchase a premade mix, you simply must have a really good all-purpose mixture on hand at all times . . . and a lot of it! Try out my recipe for yourself; experiment with others, and don't give up until you find one—any one—that you like.

Although you certainly can mix up just one simple recipe of flour (1 part = 1 cup), which will result in 4 cups of wonderful flour to use for any type of recipe, if I am going to bother lining up six ingredients and a large mixing bowl, I make several times this quantity at one time.

Another tip I'll share is to use gallon-size resealable plastic bags to do the actual mixing, in lieu of mixing bowls. Measure and pour your flour ingredi-

Jules's Nearly Normal All-Purpose Flour Mix

1 part fine white rice flour

1 part potato starch (not potato flour)

1 part cornstarch

$1/2$ part fine corn flour

$1/2$ part tapioca starch

1 teaspoon xanthan gum per cup of flour mix

Handy Substitutions for Other Food Allergies

If you have additional food allergies and cannot tolerate one of the ingredients in my mix, try these substitutions. (See Month 12 for more options with alternative flours.)

Ingredient	Substitution
Corn flour	almond flour, bean flour, or chestnut flour
Cornstarch	arrowroot or increase the tapioca starch proportion to cover the cornstarch proportion as well
Potato starch	arrowroot or increase the tapioca starch proportion to cover the potato starch proportion
Tapioca starch	arrowroot or increase both the potato and cornstarch by one-half part each
White rice flour	sorghum flour or Montina flour

ents into the bag (sit the bag inside a large bowl for support), seal the bag, and shake, squish, and squeeze until all of the flours are mixed thoroughly. You may then leave the flour mix in the bag or pour it into an airtight canister for storage. I recommend the bag method because gluten-free flours are very light (particularly the starches). Have you ever noticed the results of dumping cornstarch into an open bowl? If you attempt to mix gluten-free flours in a bowl, the ambient particles will fly about and coat your entire kitchen with fine white powder by the time the mix is combined. Believe me, my own trials and errors developed this plastic bag system, and I'm never going back!

IN A SENTENCE

You need to begin with a plan of action, and the first step in a successful gluten-free diet plan is identifying a truly all-purpose gluten-free flour that you can depend on to use in your old favorite recipes and in any new recipes you undertake.

DAY 7

learning and living

A Simple, Healing Five-Day Meal Planner

WHILE BEING a drastic departure from your regular routine, your first days of living totally gluten-free should accomplish a few things. First, it should be easy enough to convince you that you really can do it. Second, it should be tasty enough to convince you that you really want to do it. Third, it should be made up of ingredients that will be easy on your digestive tract so that you will begin to feel better as soon as possible. And fourth, the ingredients and food should be easily obtained. With all that in mind, I have devised a five-day menu planner to assist your launch into living gluten-free.

Day 1

BREAKFAST

Fresh Fruit and
Warm Grits with Maple Syrup

ANY BRAND of corn grits without flavoring should be gluten-free. Most brands of grits are enriched, so they provide extra vitamins and minerals such as iron, folic acid, thiamine, riboflavin, and niacin, as well as offer a good source of protein and dietary fiber. Follow the package directions for stove-top or microwave cooking to make a batch sufficient for the whole family to celebrate your new gluten-free life.

Any temptation your children might have to shy away from this Southern comfort food should be tamped down by the addition of real maple syrup (what child can resist syrup?!). I recommend 100 percent maple syrup for several reasons, not the least of which is the taste! It is also not overly processed and does not contain gluten in this pure form, whereas many brands of maple syrup look-alikes actually contain some gluten and should be avoided (e.g., Mrs. Butterworth's brand).

LUNCH

Spinach and Mushroom Quesadillas

THE QUESADILLA is one of my favorite dishes because it can be prepared so many different ways yet always seems to be delicious. Be sure to use corn, not flour, tortillas, and substitute ingredients if you have sensitivities to any of those suggested below.

Dairy products, for example, often cause problems for newly diagnosed celiacs, as the ability to break down milk sugar (lactose) is reduced or eliminated at least temporarily through villous atrophy (see Month 12 for more information). Many celiacs regain their ability to produce lactase when their bodies heal on a gluten-free diet. If this problem applies to you, either eliminate the cheese ingredients, use soy cheese alternatives, or try taking lactase enzyme supplements (such as Lactaid brand).

Serves 4

2 cups uncooked brown rice

4 cups water

2 tablespoons olive or canola oil

1/2 pound fresh mushrooms (whichever type you prefer; different mushrooms provide totally different flavors)

1 small yellow onion, or 1/2 cup dried onion flakes

2 teaspoons garlic powder

1 bunch fresh spinach, well washed and cut into bite-size pieces (cooks down to approximately 3/4 cup)

8 (8-inch) corn tortillas

1/4 cup freshly grated Parmesan cheese

1/2 pound Pepper Jack cheese, thinly sliced

1 cup crumbled feta cheese (optional)

1/4 cup salsa

1/4 cup guacamole (optional)

1. Combine the rice and water in a saucepan and bring to a boil. Lower the heat to low, cover, and cook until all the water is absorbed, approximately 20 minutes. After rice is fully cooked, transfer it to a bowl and let cool.

2. Heat the oil in large skillet over high heat. While the oil is heating, trim and slice the mushrooms. Add the mushrooms and onions to the pan, and sprinkle in the garlic powder. Add the spinach. Sauté for 5 minutes, or until the onion is translucent. Set aside to cool.

3. Oil a small skillet or spray it with gluten-free cooking spray (be sure your spray does not contain flour!). Place one tortilla in the pan. Cook on one side over low heat, then spray the top side with cooking spray and sprinkle a bit of Parmesan cheese onto it before flipping over to cook the other side. Cook each side until the tortillas are slightly browned but not crunchy, 1 to 2 minutes per side. Repeat with the other tortillas so that one side of each tortilla has browned Parmesan on it and both sides are lightly cooked. (Simply cook both sides of the tortillas lightly if you are eliminating cheese from this recipe.)

4. Lay one cooked tortilla back onto the oiled skillet (Parmesan side facing the pan) and spoon onto it one-quarter each of the rice, mushroom mixture, Pepper Jack cheese, feta cheese, and salsa. Place another cooked tortilla on top of this mixture (Parmesan side facing out) and flip the quesadilla over, using a large spatula. Cook on the other side until the cheese begins to melt, 3 to 5 minutes.

5. Cut with a pizza cutter into four pie-shaped pieces and serve on individual plates garnished with guacamole and salsa.

DINNER

Crab or Shrimp Quiche with Vegetables

NOT ONLY is this quiche delicious, but it's easy to make because you don't have to worry about a crust! It's also a very forgiving recipe, so feel free to be creative. I've included several options for ingredients, but you may find others on hand that work just as well.

Serves 4 to 6

Extra-virgin olive oil

1–2 tablespoons butter or nondairy alternative
(e.g., Earth Balance Buttery Sticks)

1/2 cup sliced fresh mushrooms, zucchini, broccoli, corn,
chopped red potatoes, or other additions of your choosing

4 eggs, lightly beaten

1 cup light or fat-free sour cream, or soy alternative
(e.g., Tofutti Sour Supreme)

1 cup ricotta or small-curd cottage cheese, or nondairy
alternative*

1/4 cup rice flour or Nearly Normal All-Purpose Flour Mix (page 48)

Pinch of salt

1 teaspoon chopped fresh parsley

1 teaspoon dried oregano or basil (depending on your
choice of cheese)

2 cups mixed mozzarella, Parmesan, and Romano cheeses;
Monterey Jack; or other mild shredded cheese, or nondairy
alternative

8–12 ounces shrimp (chopped, if large) or crabmeat

---

*If you need a lactose-free or dairy-free alternative to cottage or ricotta cheese:
try Lactaid brand low-fat cottage cheese or use firm or extra-firm tofu; mash or
chop in a food processor to achieve the consistency of these cheeses.

1. Preheat the oven to 350°F. Select a large quiche dish, deep pie pan, or casserole large enough to hold all the ingredients, and grease the pan with olive oil.

2. Sauté the butter and vegetables, legumes, or mushrooms, or any combination thereof that you choose. Use less butter if you are not sautéing many vegetables.

3. Mix together the eggs, sour cream, ricotta cheese, rice flour, salt, and spices in a medium-size bowl.

4. Add the sautéed ingredients, shredded cheese, and seafood, and stir.

5. Pour mixture into the prepared baking pan. Bake for approximately 45 minutes, or until the center is no longer jiggly and a knife inserted into the center comes out clean.

Day 2

BREAKFAST

Eggs, Bacon, and/or Hash Browns

1. Fix your eggs scrambled, hard-boiled, fried—however you like them—and pair with real bacon or other breakfast meat that is gluten-free (check labels on any processed meats to ensure there is no gluten added) and/or hash brown potatoes. Such brands as Ore-Ida hash browns are typically gluten-free, but remember to check labels, as companies may change their ingredients from time to time. Or try shredding fresh potatoes, then frying them lightly in olive oil—these are cheaper and better than commercially prepared hash brown potatoes, and you'll know that the dish is gluten-free!

Lemon Chicken

THIS LIGHT chicken dish may be broiled, sautéed, or microwaved. Marinate in a covered glass dish for as long as possible before cooking, for maximum flavor.

Serves 6

2 tablespoons lemon juice

2 tablespoons white wine

2 tablespoons olive oil

1 clove garlic, minced

1 teaspoon honey or agave nectar

1 teaspoon dried oregano

$1/2$ teaspoon sea salt

$1/2$ teaspoon pepper

6 boneless, skinless chicken breast halves

Sliced lemon, for garnish

1. Combine the lemon juice, wine, 1 tablespoon of the olive oil, and the garlic, honey, oregano, salt, and pepper. Pour into a shallow glass baking dish and add the chicken, turning to coat both sides. Cover and refrigerate for at least 30 minutes.

2. *Sauté:* Heat the remaining oil in a large skillet over medium heat. Add the chicken, discarding any excess marinade. Cook on both sides until no longer pink in the middle, approximately 20 minutes total.

Microwave: Microwave on high, turning once, until chicken is no longer pink, or about 8 minutes.

Broil: Place the chicken on the broiler pan, brushing with the remaining olive oil. Turn once, broiling on high until no longer pink in the middle. Broiler times will vary with your oven and the thickness of the chicken breasts; check them after 5 minutes to be sure not to burn them.

Fish Stew

THIS MEXICAN-INSPIRED stew is heartier than you might imagine. It is amazingly fast and easy to make—perfect for those nights when you're running short on time!

Serves 6

2 diced and seeded fresh tomatoes

3/4 cup cooked fresh corn

1/2 teaspoon ground cumin

1/4 cup chopped fresh cilantro, plus extra leaves for garnish

1 pound new potatoes, washed and sliced

1–2 large shallots or small sweet onions (e.g., Vidalia), peeled and thinly sliced, or to taste

1 teaspoon extra-virgin olive oil

1 teaspoon sea salt

1/2 teaspoon coarsely ground pepper

1 pound skinless cod, grouper, or red snapper fillet, cut into 1 1/2-inch chunks

Pinch of red pepper flakes

1 cup cooked brown or white rice (optional)

1. Mix together the tomatoes, corn, cumin, and cilantro in a medium-size bowl and set aside.

2. Combine the sliced potatoes and shallots and oil in a 2-quart microwave-safe dish. Stir to distribute the oil, then arrange the potatoes and shallots in an even layer and sprinkle half of the salt and pepper over the top. Cover and microwave on high for 5 to 6 minutes, depending on how thinly the potatoes are sliced.

3. Arrange the fish chunks in a single layer around the outside of the dish, on top of the potatoes. Season with the remaining salt and pepper (add the red pepper here if you want extra spice).

4. Pour the vegetable mixture into the middle of the dish. Cover again and microwave on high until the fish and potatoes are cooked through, 9 to 10 minutes.

5. Stir to combine everything. If using cooked rice, stir into the cooked stew or pour the stew over each serving of the rice; if not using rice, spoon the stew into bowls and garnish with fresh cilantro leaves.

Old-Fashioned Rice Pudding

THIS RECIPE calls for pearl, or pudding, rice, which is available at most organic or health food stores. It makes a traditional British form of rice pudding, to which you can add cinnamon, raisins, cranberries, or any other addition you find yummy. It is definitely a feel-good food and makes even a cold rainy day seem a little better. Try it for breakfast or for dessert!

Serves 4

3 tablespoons short-grain pudding rice

2^1/2 cups milk (dairy, rice, almond, coconut, or soy)

1 tablespoon honey or agave nectar

^{1}/2 teaspoon gluten-free vanilla extract

1 tablespoon butter or nondairy alternative

^{1}/2 cup seedless raisins, cranberries, or other additions of your choice

1. Preheat the oven to 300°F. Grease or butter a shallow baking dish.

2. Mix the rice, milk, honey, and vanilla extract together in a bowl. Pour into the greased baking dish and dot the top of the mixture with butter.

3. Bake for 30 minutes, then stir the skin into the pudding.

4. Bake for 1^1/2 to 2 hours more, again stirring the skin into the pudding every 30 minutes. Stir in the raisins or other additions and reduce the oven temperature to 250°F after 1 full hour of baking.

5. Remove from the oven when the pudding is set through.

Day 3

BREAKFAST

Fluffy Omelet

THIS DISH is great for breakfast or dinner, depending on what you pair with it.

Serves 2

4 eggs

2 tablespoons water

1 tablespoon butter or nondairy alternative

1. Preheat the oven to 325°F.

2. Separate the eggs into two separate bowls, putting the whites in a large ceramic or metal bowl, and the yolks into a small bowl.

3. Beat the yolks lightly and set aside.

4. Beat the egg whites with a clean mixer attachment until fluffy. Add the water and continue beating for about 1 1/2 minutes longer, or until stiff peaks form. Gently fold the egg yolks into the egg whites.

5. Heat the butter in a large ovenproof skillet, and pour the egg mixture into the middle, spreading it with slightly higher sides. Cook on the stove top over low heat for 8 to 10 minutes, or until it is fluffy and is lightly browned on the bottom.

6. Remove from the stove top and put into the oven for another 8 to 10 minutes, or until a knife inserted into the center is clean. Loosen the sides of the omelet from the pan and make a shallow cut slightly off center across the middle of the omelet. Fold the smaller side over the larger side and serve warm.

7. If you want to add cheese or sautéed vegetables to the omelet, add the warmed ingredients just before folding over. Otherwise, serve with maple syrup for a delicious and filling breakfast!

LUNCH

Fresh Grilled Fish

CHOOSE YOUR favorite fish, fillet, and grill—nothing difficult, just delicious! I recommend a white fish such as mahimahi for this easy preparation.

Fish fillets

Extra-virgin olive oil

Sea salt and fresh ground pepper

Tomato salsa (optional)

1. Clean your grill and brush with olive oil or line with foil coated with olive oil. Heat to medium-high.

2. Brush the fish fillets with olive oil and season lightly with salt and pepper.

3. Grill 3 to 4 minutes per side (longer if thicker pieces), turning gently with a large oiled spatula.

4. Remove from the heat when the fish is opaque throughout and flakes easily with a fork.

5. Serve immediately as is, or with fresh tomato salsa on top.

Greek Mashed Potatoes

THIS RECIPE makes wonderful mashed potatoes, whether or not you choose to add the Greek flavoring.

Serves 4

3 baking potatoes, peeled and cut into 2-inch chunks

Sea salt and freshly ground pepper

Cold water, or homemade or commercially available gluten-free vegetable or chicken stock

1 cup milk (dairy, rice, almond, coconut, or soy)

4 ounces feta cheese (optional)

2 thinly sliced fresh scallions, leeks, or shallots

1. Mix the potato chunks, salt, and enough water or stock to measure 2 inches deep in a large saucepan. Boil over medium-high heat.

2. Reduce the heat to medium after the mixture boils and simmer for approximately 15 minutes, or until the potatoes are tender but not mushy.

3. Drain the potatoes and return them to the saucepan.

4. Cook over medium heat while adding the milk and feta cheese until warmed through.

5. Remove from the heat and mash the mixture together, using a potato masher, until it is the consistency you prefer for your mashed potatoes.

6. Season with additional salt and pepper and stir in the scallions.

7. Serve warm.

Lemon-Oregano Herb-Rubbed Chicken Breasts

THESE CHICKEN breasts can be cooked in a skillet or on the grill. The chicken should be "rubbed" at least two hours in advance, longer if possible. Also, the breasts can be rubbed with the spices and then frozen, so all you have to do for dinner is thaw and cook.

Serves 4

Rub

2 cloves garlic, pressed

1 tablespoon lemon pepper

1 tablespoon olive oil

1$^{1}/_{2}$ teaspoons dried oregano

4 chicken breasts

Additional olive oil, if stir-frying

Vegetables, such as carrots, squash, onions, and peppers

Cooked rice, if stir-frying

1. In a small bowl, mix together all the rub ingredients. Wearing kitchen gloves, rub mixture onto both sides of the chicken breasts.

2. *Grill:* Grill both sides of the breasts until the chicken is no longer pink in the middle.

Stir-fry: Cut into bite-size strips and stir-fry in a large skillet or wok in additional olive oil with vegetables for 8 to 10 minutes, being careful not to overcook, then serve over rice.

Day 4

BREAKFAST

Potato Omelet

A HEARTY meal—yes, meal—that serves four.

$1/3$ cup ($5^1/3$ tablespoons) butter or nondairy alternative

2 medium-size baking potatoes, peeled and finely chopped

$1/4$ cup sliced onion

6 eggs

2 tablespoons milk or nondairy alternative

Salt and pepper

1 cup diced cooked chicken (optional)

1. Heat the butter in a large skillet and add the potatoes and onion. Turning often, cook until tender, 8 to 10 minutes.

2. Beat together the eggs, milk, salt, and pepper (add chicken here if using) in a medium-size bowl.

3. Pour over the cooked potatoes and cook without stirring until the mixture begins to set. Lift the edges of the omelet and tilt the pan to allow any uncooked eggs to run underneath and contact the hot pan. Cook until the eggs are dry enough to suit your taste and cut the omelets into portions to serve on individual plates.

Nutty Rice

THIS RECIPE is a great one to start and forget in a slow cooker while you move on to bigger projects. It is a great reward to come back to, offering hearty protein, fiber, and taste. You can add any leftover chicken or fish from other days to make the dish a more filling meal.

Serves 4

2/3 cup raw nuts (cashews, peanuts, walnuts, or almonds)

1/3 cup water

1 1/3 cups homemade chicken stock or vegetable broth

1 cup uncooked quick/instant brown rice

1/4 teaspoon salt

1/8 teaspoon ground turmeric

1. In a blender or food processor, blend 1/3 cup of the raw nuts and 1/3 cup of water. Pour the mixture into your slow cooker or a stove-top pot.

2. Stir in the remaining ingredients. Cook in the slow cooker for 1 1/2 to 2 hours, or until the rice is soft. If using a stove-top pot, bring to a boil, then lower the heat to a simmer, covering with a tight-fitting lid and stirring occasionally, cooking until the rice is soft throughout, 25 to 30 minutes.

DINNER

Black Bean Quesadillas

ANOTHER ROUND of totally different quesadillas that are quick and easy to make and will satisfy your taste buds!

Serves 8

1 (15-ounce) can black beans, rinsed and drained

$1/2$ cup chunky salsa

$1/4$ cup sweet corn kernels

1 ($1/4$-ounce) packet Sazón Goya seasoning or gluten-free taco seasoning*

$1/2$ pound Pepper Jack, mozzarella, Cheddar, or a mixture of dairy or nondairy cheeses, shredded

$1/4$ cup guacamole (optional)

8 (8-inch) corn tortillas

1. In a saucepan over medium heat, combine all ingredients except for the cheese, guacamole, and tortillas. Stir to mix, cover, and heat until the mixture is cooked through but not boiling. Remove from the heat and set aside.

2. Oil a small skillet or spray it with gluten-free cooking spray (be sure your spray does not contain flour!). Place one tortilla in the pan. Cook on one side over low heat until lightly browned, then turn and cook the other side. Cook until the tortilla is slightly browned but not crunchy, 1 to 2 minutes per side. Repeat with the other tortillas.

3. Lay one cooked tortilla back onto the oiled skillet and spoon one-quarter of the bean mixture and the cheese on top. Place another cooked tortilla on top of this mixture. Turn over the quesadilla, using a large spatula, and cook on the other side until the cheese begins to melt.

4. Serve on individual plates, garnished with guacamole and salsa. Add rice as a side dish, if desired.

---

*If you cannot find any commercially available gluten-free taco seasoning, try this easy mixture:

1 teaspoon chile powder

$1/2$ teaspoon salt

$1/2$ teaspoon black pepper

$1/2$ teaspoon garlic powder

$1/2$ teaspoon ground cumin

Homemade Applesauce

ALTHOUGH THE finished product will be better than any you could buy in a store, this recipe is deceptively simple and pure! Choose naturally sweet apples like Gala, Fuji, Rome, or Red Delicious (avoid sour apples such as Granny Smith, which require the addition of sugar) and always mix up your choices rather than using only one type of apple.

> Apples (3 to 4 pounds per quart of cooked applesauce)
> Water
> Ground cinnamon (optional)

1. Wash the apples in cold water and peel them, using a vegetable peeler or paring knife. Remove any hard sections, including the core and seeds, then chop to a uniformly small size to suit your taste. You can use larger chunks if you prefer chunkier applesauce.

2. Fill a large heavy-bottomed saucepan or stockpot with 1 inch of water. Add the apples and cover with a tight-fitting lid. Heat the apples and water over high heat until boiling, then lower the heat to medium and cook until the apples are soft. Stir periodically to keep them from sticking to the bottom and to test for doneness.

3. If you have a sieve or strainer, pour the apples through the sieve; otherwise, stir the softened apples vigorously in the pot until they are the mushy consistency you prefer for your applesauce. (A potato masher or whisk works nicely if you do not have a sieve or strainer.) If you like very smooth applesauce, you can put the cooked apples into a food processor or blender to puree.

4. At this point, you can enjoy the pure taste of fresh applesauce naturally (or you may add cinnamon)! It should stay fresh in your refrigerator for approximately 2 weeks, or you may freeze or can it (if you can refrain from eating it all right away!).

Day 5

BREAKFAST

Tropical Rice

THIS RECIPE will definitely awaken taste buds you didn't think you had. Try it as a cereal for a total change of pace by adding milk or additional pineapple juice.

Serves 4

1 cup crushed fresh pineapple

1/2 cup fresh pineapple juice (from the crushed pineapple)

3/4 cup brown rice

1/4 cup chopped or slivered raw almonds

1/2 teaspoon salt

1/2 cup dried raisins or cranberries

1. Place all ingredients (except for the dried fruit) in a slow cooker or stove-top pot.

2. In the slow cooker, cook until the rice is soft, approximately 5 hours; on the stove-top, bring to a boil, stirring, then quickly lower the heat to a simmer, cover with a tight-fitting lid, and cook until the rice is softened, 20 to 25 minutes.

3. Turn off the slow cooker or stove-top heat as soon as the rice is cooked, then stir in the dried fruit.

4. Let stand for 5 minutes.

5. Serve warm, adding milk or additional pineapple juice to thin for morning cereal, or serving as is with fish or chicken.

Vegetable Frittata

THIS FILLING dish is akin to an open-faced omelet and serves approximately three people. It is very forgiving (my favorite kind of recipe!), so add whatever ingredients you have on hand.

> 6 eggs
> Salt and pepper
> 1 tablespoon butter or nondairy alternative
> 1 clove garlic, minced
> 1 cup chopped fresh vegetables of your choice (such as yellow squash, zucchini, broccoli, peppers, onions, and/or mushrooms)
> 2 tablespoons grated Parmesan or Romano cheese, or nondairy alternative (optional)

1. Preheat the oven by turning on the broiler.

2. Beat the eggs, salt, and pepper together in a medium-size bowl and set aside.

3. In a 10-inch ovenproof skillet, melt the butter and stir in the garlic and onions (if using) until tender. Next, stir in your other vegetables and sauté until tender.

4. Pour the mixed eggs over the vegetables in the skillet. Tilt the pan and lift the sides of the eggs as they set, to allow the uncooked eggs to contact the hot pan. Continue cooking until the eggs are nearly set and but not yet dry.

5. Place the ovenproof skillet under the broiler, 4 to 5 inches from the heat source. Broil just until the top is set—1 to 2 minutes.

6. Remove from the heat and sprinkle with the cheese. Cut into wedges to serve.

DINNER

Sweet Shrimp

THIS RECIPE is handy for entertaining, as the dressing may be made up to a week in advance and the entire dish prepared the night before. Serve with any leftover rice or potatoes you have from other meals.

Serves 4

Dressing

 1 teaspoon mustard seeds

 1 teaspoon ground cinnamon

 2 tablespoons fresh lemon juice

 4 tablespoons honey or agave nectar

 $1/2$ cup apple cider vinegar

 2 teaspoons dry mustard

 2 tablespoons fresh dill

 2 tablespoons finely chopped red onion

 $1/2$ cup vegetable oil

 2 pounds medium-size shrimp, cooked

1. Toast the mustard seeds on a cookie sheet under the broiler for 1 to 2 minutes, until they start popping like popcorn.

2. In a bowl, combine all the other dressing ingredients with the toasted mustard seeds and whisk in the oil. Chill, tightly covered, in a jar (keeps for about a week).

3. At least 2 hours before serving, mix the cooked shrimp with the dressing.

4. Refrigerate for at least 2 hours. Serve over rice or potatoes for a meal.

IN A SENTENCE

> *With these recipes, you can begin your journey to gluten-free living with confidence and relative ease and know that it is not only possible to cook and eat gluten-free but actually very manageable and tasty.*

FIRST-WEEK MILESTONE

You have had a lot to take in this first week, but tackling it one piece at a time will allow you to learn and adjust in manageable increments. You have learned:

○ ALL ABOUT THE FOOD PROTEIN GLUTEN, WHERE IT IS FOUND, AND WHAT FOODS ARE SAFE TO EAT BECAUSE THEY ARE NATURALLY GLUTEN-FREE

○ HOW CELIAC DISEASE HURTS OUR BODIES FROM THE INSIDE OUT, THE IMPORTANCE OF TESTING FOR CELIAC DISEASE, AND HOW THOSE TESTS ARE ADMINISTERED

○ THE NATURAL TENDENCY TO DOUBT A LIFE-CHANGING DIAGNOSIS, AS WELL AS THE UN-AVOIDABLE INITIAL FEELINGS OF BEING OVERWHELMED

○ THAT YOU CAN TAKE CHARGE OF YOUR HEALTH WITHOUT RELYING ON PRESCRIP-TION MEDICINES OR INVASIVE TREATMENT TECHNIQUES

○ HOW TO BEGIN A NEW GLUTEN-FREE LIFE WITH AN ALL-PURPOSE GLUTEN-FREE FLOUR MIX AND HEALTHY, EASY, AND DELICIOUS RECIPES

Your New Gluten-Free Kitchen in Seven Easy Steps

THROUGHOUT THE next several weeks, you will learn in depth how to successfully and easily adapt your kitchen, your cooking, and your habits to live gluten-free. The first step is to incorporate significant changes in the kitchen. This chapter provides seven tips to get you on the gluten-free road quickly and easily. Each step is crucial in your transition to a gluten-free life. Take the time to do it right from the beginning; a good base will alleviate some of the stress and confusion.

Before we get started, though, it is important to understand just why a fresh beginning is so essential. Your doctor may have explained that gluten contamination is a serious concern. This is not just true of factories where grains and other food products are processed or packaged. Your own kitchen may well be the biggest culprit if you are not deliberate in your cross-contamination prevention.

By now you understand how damaging gluten can be to anyone with celiac disease. But you must realize that even dust or crumbs of a gluten-containing food can cause such problems if they find their way into your meal. As mentioned earlier, even consuming as little as $1/8$ teaspoon of gluten can damage your intestine. Never simply pick the croutons off a salad or eat just the filling removed from a prepared sandwich, and never risk using condiments and spreads; pots and pans; cutting boards and utensils; or appliances that may have even a trace of remains from a non-gluten-free food. These types of avoidance techniques will go a long way toward protecting you and other gluten-free family members from accidental gluten contamination. Read on for specific tips to clean, prepare, and reorganize your new gluten-free kitchen.

1. Clean Out and Reorganize Your Pantry

Most of us could use a good old-fashioned spring cleaning in the pantry anyway, so use this occasion as a kick in the pants to get you moving. Sit down with a big cardboard box and a trash bag. Put all the foods that contain gluten into the box; put all the things that are expired or open into the trash bag. Now review the items that contain gluten. What are you really sad to see go? Make a list—next week we'll go shopping to buy a gluten-free substitute (or you can use a recipe to make it yourself!). Take the box of gluten-containing products to your local homeless shelter or food bank and pat yourself on the back: you have now done a good thing for yourself and for others.

To make sure that the pantry is entirely gluten-free, thoroughly clean the surfaces of these cabinets and shelves, ensuring that not so much as a speck from the last bag of flour or box of cereal could find its way into your special gluten-free foods. If you plan to reuse containers that once contained non-gluten-free foods, give them a good scrubbing, especially along any seams and under the rims.

If anyone in your family is not going gluten-free, you'll need to designate separate sections or cabinets in the pantry to store your gluten-free items in as airtight a manner as you can, and that includes inside the fridge. Within your refrigerator and freezer, enclose in tightly lidded containers or sealed plastic bags any item that contains gluten, so that crumbs or other matter cannot transfer by accident to the other foods stored nearby.

Label the gluten-free sections with stickers, colorful tape, or whatever creative ideas you and your family can devise that celebrate these dedicated areas or packages as being yummy and fun. Believe me, when we're done, they will be both. And, you will want to celebrate that you and your family can eat good, safe, and healthy food again, together!

2. Buy a New Toaster

If you have ever tried to clean a toaster—I mean *really* clean a toaster—you know that it is nearly impossible to remove every last crumb. Make the inexpensive investment in a new toaster and some peace of mind. If there are gluten eaters in your household, dedicate this new toaster to only gluten-free foods and attach a fun sticker or colored electrical tape to the toaster for a friendly reminder!

3. No Double-Dipping

If possible, use condiments that come from squeeze bottles. Otherwise, have a house rule that there is only one dip into a jar or tub with any given utensil. Bread crumbs can stick to the peanut butter on a knife and return to sit in a jar until the next unsuspecting person digs in—don't let it be you!

4. Replace Pans with Worn Surfaces

Many people suggest that you buy all new pans when you go gluten-free, and that you have dedicated pans and utensils for gluten-free items. If this is possible with your budget and your kitchen storage space, then great. However, for most of us, an entirely new kitchen set (and finding somewhere separate to store it, if you are also keeping your present equipment to use for non-gluten-free preparation) is not necessarily a viable option. Instead, thoroughly examine any pots and pans for worn surfaces, crusted seams and rims, and/or scratches or dents that could harbor food between meals. It is probably time to replace these anyway, and going gluten-free is the perfect excuse. If you can separate out any cookware for dedicated gluten-free use, more power to you. I often recommend to my clients that they identify these pots with brightly colored electrical tape wrapped around the handles! If you simply cannot dedicate pans to be exclusively used for gluten-free fare, then be sure to always wash all items in a dishwasher, using the entire series of washing and drying cycles to ensure that the pans are truly cleaned.

Take particular care with grills, grates, and racks, which are notoriously hard to clean even if one doesn't need to avoid gluten—all those tiny joints and holes are a perpetual trap for sticky substances. At the very least, if you plan to bake breads or desserts, invest in a dedicated gluten-free cake cooling rack. If your outdoor grill or oven grates have ever been used for foods with breaded coatings or marinades, or bread products have been placed directly on a grate for toasting, see if you can buy an extra grate to be used only for gluten-free foods. If not, scrub the old grate as thoroughly as you can before each use, and cook your own meal first before grilling anyone else's food that could cross-contaminate the grate's complex surfaces.

5. Become an Avid Label Reader

If you are anything like me, you are so busy that you don't have time to read anything longer than a label. So go ahead and read those labels! When you clean your pantry, use the opportunity to become accustomed to label terminology and other names for potential gluten sources, such as malt flavoring, brown rice syrup, malt vinegar, or any unspecified thickeners, stabilizers, starches, or flavorings. By the time you have reorganized your pantry, you will be an expert label reader and can fly down the market aisles buying foods that you can trust to eat! Carry lists of gluten-free grains and gluten-containing ingredients so that you have a reference to double-check, in case you run across something new or unique. You don't need to spend money to obtain these lists; there is plenty of free information on the Internet, and you can even carry along this book or photocopy the lists on pages 19, 20, and 24. As you discover them, jot down the names of manufacturers dedicated to gluten-free products, so that you can easily spot them while shopping in markets where gluten-free items are integrated into the shelves of conventional foods.

6. Mix or Buy a Big Batch of All-Purpose Gluten-Free Flour

When you are cooking or baking gluten-free, one of the hardest things to get used to is that the list of dry ingredients is usually double that of most ordinary recipes. Don't let that deter you! As described last week (page 48), one of the easiest tips for your new gluten-free kitchen is to either buy a big bag of your favorite all-purpose gluten-free flour or mix a large batch and store it in your cupboard. If the flour is ready to go, you have probably just cut the dry ingredients list and preparation time of your gluten-free recipe in half, and you certainly have cut back on possible excuses not to bake!

On Day 6 you learned how to make your own all-purpose gluten-free flour. This product is truly the one essential ingredient to living gluten-free (there are many other useful things that I will discuss, but this one is crucial). I will introduce you to different kinds of all-purpose flours in week 3 when we go shopping, but for now, mark your shopping list with an asterisk next to "ingredients necessary to make your own flour" or "buy gluten-free flours." While you are making your list, be sure to also add a note to purchase several new tightly lidded containers in which to store your flour, mixes, and snacks, to keep them fresh and isolated from any other gluten-containing foods that you may decide to keep around for other members of your family.

How to Contact Food Manufacturers to Check If a Food Product Is Gluten-Free

Many companies' food labels list no gluten-containing ingredients, yet they do not use the term "gluten-free" on their containers. As the food labeling laws come into effect, this situation will be less and less prevalent, nevertheless, it is useful to consider what you as a gluten-free consumer should do when confronted with these products. When there is no indication on the packaging or the company Web site that the product is indeed gluten-free, you should investigate further. Do not simply assume that the product has been manufactured in a gluten-free environment, or that any additives are gluten-free. You may call or write to the company and you should expect to receive confirmation one way or the other, which will help you to make a determination of how that product may fit into your dietary restrictions. I have included a response I received from one such investigation so that you may know what kind of explanation you can expect to receive. In this case, the company seemed sufficiently vigilant about trace gluten for me to trust that its products whose labels did not list gluten as an ingredient were indeed gluten-free.

Dear Ms. Shepard,

Thank you for taking the time to contact us regarding our product. We strive to maintain the highest quality products and appreciate your patronage.

We consider gluten to be in the following, barley, bulgur, couscous, durum, graham flour, kamut, malt, rye, semolina, spelt, triticale, and any other types of

continues

wheat. We do not consider any oat products to be gluten-free due to the fact that studies are needed to determine the long-term safety of oat consumption. The issue of cross contamination with oat and wheat remains a concern in North America.

We do not have lists of products that are specifically considered to be gluten-free. Reading the label is the best way to check for the presence of ingredients which contain gluten. If gluten is an ingredient, it is listed separately and not under "natural flavors" or "spices." Consumer health and safety is our number one concern, and we do not want to provide information which may not be accurate in the future.

Our company's labeling declares major allergens (peanuts, soybeans, milk, eggs, fish, crustaceans, tree nuts, and wheat) and we follow the U.S. FDA's regulations. In addition, our labeling always declares gluten-containing ingredients. We recognize the serious nature of the allergen issue and we strive to minimize risk.

Both major and minor ingredients of all products, as well as all processing procedures and equipment, are closely scrutinized and all potential allergen issues as determined by our company are declared on our labeling.

We assure you that strict manufacturing processes and procedures are in place and that all of our manufacturing facilities follow rigid allergen control programs that include staff training, segregation of allergen ingredients, production scheduling, and thorough cleaning and sanitation.

Thank you for your continued support. If we can be of further assistance, please feel free to contact us Monday through Friday from 7 a.m.–5 p.m.

Sincerely,
Kathy
Consumer Relations

7. Limit Gluten in the Kitchen

If you have any members of your household who are not already gluten-free, then they should now eat gluten-free meals with you. I understand buying your non-gluten-free child occasional gluten-containing items, such as regular sandwich bread to pack for a school lunch (who wants to waste good gluten-free bread on a sandwich your child might not even eat, since you aren't there to make sure he or she eats the sandwich *before* the pudding?!). But there is honestly no reason why you should have any gluten flour in your kitchen anymore. You will soon be armed with the information necessary to make great gluten-free food everyone can enjoy . . . together!

It is cheaper, easier, more efficient, and more conducive to family dining if you can all enjoy the same foods and lick the bowl together. Once everyone tastes the delicious and easy dishes available on your diet, there will be no excuses! Furthermore, one of the easiest ways to stay on a gluten-free diet is to have the support of your family and friends. If your family eats different food at every meal, it will be much harder for you to stay on a gluten-free diet and to remain positive about your new lifestyle.

Your New Gluten-Free Kitchen in Seven Easy Steps

1. Clean out and reorganize your pantry.
2. Buy a new toaster.
3. No double-dipping.
4. Replace pans with worn surfaces.
5. Become an avid label reader.
6. Mix or buy a big batch of all-purpose gluten-free flour.
7. Limit gluten in the kitchen.

IN A SENTENCE

Adapting your kitchen to these new cooking and eating habits is the first big step to take on the road to your new gluten-free life and good health.

WEEK **3**

learning and living

Shopping Gluten-Free in Six Easy Steps

NOW THAT you've cleaned out your kitchen, grab your pen and paper and let's get ready to shop! This is the fun part, but it can also be quite daunting. You will be shocked at how many gluten-free products are actually on the market, with more entering your supermarket and organic grocery each day. The gluten-free market—a $210 million industry in 2001—is projected to be a $1.7 billion market by 2010![1] Food manufacturers are starting to notice the need and they are scrambling to fill it. Only some of these companies have done a good job of filling the need with truly tasty options, though. The purpose of this chapter is to prepare you for how to replace the essentials in your pantry with gluten-free versions, and to arm you with the information necessary to pick and choose amongst the options in everything else.

---

1. Packaged Facts, "Gluten-Free Foods and Beverages in the U.S.," (July 1, 2006).

Create a Shopping List

1. CHOOSE AN ALL-PURPOSE GLUTEN-FREE
FLOUR MIXTURE OR RECIPE

When you cook or bake, you'll need a good flour to substitute for gluten-containing all-purpose wheat flour.

The gluten-free all-purpose flour mix that will get you through the first year of living gluten-free, if not through the rest of your gluten-free adventures thereafter, is one that should not have too high a proportion of gritty grain ingredients such as rice flour, and it must have enough starchy lighteners to keep your recipes from being too dense and heavy.

If you choose to make your own all-purpose mixture, understand that you will be shopping for enough ingredients to make a large quantity of this mix. You do not want to feel as if you cannot bake something simply because you do not have enough or do not want to use it all up on a particular recipe. The idea is to make your life as similar to the way it was before you were baking gluten-free. Thus, when you pick up a recipe to make for dinner, you will simply scoop out the required measurement of gluten-free flour mix as you would have when you used a wheat-based flour. Especially if you are less than confident in the kitchen, you need to eliminate as many steps in a recipe as possible, so heed this advice. As far as your shopping list goes, you should either buy at least five to ten pounds of all-purpose premixed gluten-free flour, or add all the ingredients for your chosen recipe to your list and multiply the proportions by five or ten so that you have enough to last for a while.[2]

If you elect to purchase a premade all-purpose mix (the much easier, although not necessarily always cheaper option), ensure that the mix you choose already includes a binder, such as xanthan gum. You will learn on your first trip to the store that xanthan and guar gums are by far the most expensive ingredient in any gluten-free flour mix. Why should you buy a

---

2. Unless you are using flours with a high fat content, most gluten-free flours should not need to be refrigerated (more on these flours in Month 12) and can be stored tightly sealed in a cool, dark cabinet for around a year or so.

so-called all-purpose mix and be expected to also have to buy, measure, and add the most expensive ingredient yourself? You shouldn't. Armed with these shopping hints, you will be able to select or make a truly all-purpose mixture from your first big trip to the store.

At least in the beginning of your new gluten-free life, you should stick to a tried and true recipe or premade mix that allows you to make anything you want to make quickly and successfully. Later, if and when you have the inclination, feel free to experiment with other gluten-free flour options and make your own mixes tailored to your tastes and dietary needs. I get into the details of these ingredient options in Month 12, when we go over advanced gluten-free baking, but for now, concern yourself only with finding a good mixture, not with understanding the intricacies of each potential ingredient.

2. PICK YOUR FAVORITE SNACKS

Next on your list should be all the things you liked to munch on between meals before you were eating gluten-free.

For example, if you like to eat fruit, peanuts, potato chips, popcorn, and pretzels, then you will be shopping for gluten-free varieties of all of these items.

Fruit is naturally gluten-free, so nothing would change here.

Peanuts are also gluten-free, unless you buy some specially roasted varieties in which they add wheat starch or other glutenous flavorings; here you would simply have to read the labels or choose plain salted or unsalted nuts.

Many, if not most, potato chips are already gluten-free. Simple is best here as well, since flavorings are the place where gluten often lurks. Check Web sites and labels to ensure your brands are gluten-free, paying particular attention to chips in unnatural shapes, such as Pringles chips, which use wheat starch to hold their shapes. One rice chip option that offers numerous delicious flavors is Mr. Krispers.

Popcorn is naturally gluten-free, unless additional flavorings are used that are made with gluten.

Pretzels are the only snack on this list for which you will probably need to shop at a specialty food store. Typical store brands are all made using wheat flour, so you will need to look to gluten-free specialty brands currently only available at organic food markets and online retailers. Fortunately, gluten-free pretzels have evolved to the point that they are delicious and interchangeable with wheat varieties for any social occasion. For my money,

Glutino sticks and twists taste the best and are the best buy (they even come in family-size 14-ounce packages).[3]

3. IDENTIFY MEAL INGREDIENTS

Next, you will want to consider meal options. I recommend having a few frozen dishes on hand for emergencies, such as gluten-free fish sticks, frozen gluten-free bagels, gluten-free pasta meals such as macaroni and cheese or tuna noodle casserole, and so on. As you get used to the diet, you will find other things that you particularly enjoy and you want to keep those on hand at all times. Supplement with experimental choices and ingredients for new recipes. Your own kitchen is your refuge and your fallback for times when you are concerned about gluten contamination or just want to be confident that you always have something available to eat. Make sure it is well stocked with foods that bring you comfort and happiness.

Breakfast.   For breakfast, add some gluten-free cereals to your list, perhaps instant grits or gluten-free oats, gluten-free frozen waffles, maple syrup, yogurt, and fresh fruit.

Lunch.   Lunch begins to get more complicated, as there are so many more options. You will need some handy sides, such as the snacks we covered earlier. Other options that are great for children's lunches include many readymade puddings, gelatin desserts, yogurts, and applesauce. Many trail mixes, raisins, and other dried or cut fruits make good accompaniments for a lunch box as well. Nearly all (unprocessed) cheeses, jellies, and peanut butters are gluten-free, so you can rest easy there (although you should always doublecheck labels), and you must confirm that any processed lunch meats are free of added glutens.

---

3. Throughout the book, I may periodically reference particular brands of gluten-free foods. I recommend these brands because, as this book is written, they are gluten-free, I have tasted and/or used them myself, and they taste good. I believe that part of the challenge of initially learning to live gluten-free is that you have to discern which products are worth buying, and I hope my recommendations will help to save you time and money. I have not been paid by any manufacturer to endorse their products; I simply offer you my personal recommendations that you can accept or ignore. Please do not forget to actually confirm that every product you purchase is gluten-free, as companies frequently change recipes, ingredients, and suppliers.

If you like to pack a sandwich for lunch every day, then finding a good gluten-free bread will be a priority for you. Making your own bread is always the best way to go to get really good, fresh, and delicious bread; however, that option might not be realistic for you. If not, then look to see if there is a bakery or natural foods store nearby that carries gluten-free bread—the next best option. Otherwise, you will probably be searching for the best frozen options; if this is the case, you should investigate the various online gluten-free forums. Sales outlets such as www.glutenfreemall.com and Listservs (more on these in Week 4 on support groups) post other purchasers' opinions about products. Some good brands to look for are Dr. Schar, Foods by George, Glutano, Josefs, and Kinnikinnick (which also makes very good frozen gluten-free bagels!). Gluten-free wraps or corn tortillas are other options for lunch sandwiches. Individual manufacturers' Web sites may offer an option to ship fresh bread to you as well, so check around for those choices.

Dinner.   What about dinner? What meals does your family most enjoy eating? What meals are already gluten-free? For example, my kids and I had homemade tacos and fruit salad at my house this evening. Everything we made was already gluten-free: taco filling (we just had to double-check that the seasoning we used was gluten-free), shredded Cheddar cheese, salsa, lettuce, tomatoes, corn taco shells, and fruit. If there are other meals you particularly enjoy, you need to identify them and add them to your list to find gluten-free options at the store. Start out simple with things, such as substituting store-bought gluten-free pasta noodles (most grocery stores now carry some brands—I like Tinkyáda and Mrs. Leeper's brands best) with your favorite pasta sauce (most are already gluten-free), rather than diving in to attempt a homemade gluten-free pizza. All recipes are possible to render gluten-free, and you will master what you want to master in time; for now, though, you need to make your learning curve as manageable as possible.

For those who have never had the time or the inclination to prepare homemade foods, I understand that these suggestions may seem off the mark for you. The same advice holds true for your eating habits as well. Look to your own typical eating habits and try to replace them with the same sorts of gluten-free options. For example, if you are a frozen dinner fan, there are some great gluten-free options from such brands as Amy's Kitchen, which are readily available in both health food stores and many regular grocery stores as well. If you would prefer to have fresh dinners delivered to your door, such companies as PurFoods Gluten-Free Foods (www.glutenfreemeals.com) can fill that need with full meal plans or single-order meals. Whatever your tastes, more and more companies are cropping up to fill it, so never fear, your gluten-free meal needs can be met!

4. ADD SOME COOKING ESSENTIALS

You will want to add some essentials to your list to be sure you have these around. Choose a few meals you would like to make every week or so, and keep those ingredients on your regular shopping list: rice; gluten-free pasta; pasta sauce; fresh vegetables; fresh meat, chicken, or fish; salad ingredients; ice cream; applesauce; and the like. If you enjoy particular types of foods like salads, be sure to have a good gluten-free dressing in your refrigerator. If you really like Asian foods, seek out a gluten-free soy sauce, Thai peanut sauce, or any other condiments you would like to have to spice up your meals. Again, you need to consider your typical meal and baking habits, but I would suggest including at least the following basics on your list if they are not already in your pantry or refrigerator and they otherwise fit into your dietary tastes:

Cheese (unprocessed)	Gluten-free seasoning (e.g., taco
Cornmeal	seasoning, seafood seasoning,
Corn tortillas	steak sauce, salad dressings)
Eggs	Gluten-free vanilla extract
Fresh fruit and vegetables, meat,	Oils (canola and olive)
or seafood	Pure maple syrup
Gluten-free baking powder	Rice (unflavored brown or white)
Gluten-free mashed potato flakes	Xanthan gum or guar gum

Where and How to Shop

5. CHOOSE YOUR SHOPPING VENUE

Now that you have your list of essentials, you need to evaluate your shopping options. Do you have a market nearby where you could reasonably shop for all of your list, or will you need to drive a long distance or perhaps visit several stores to finish your shopping? If you have these latter circumstances or if you are short on shopping time and prefer to shop online, there are several good choices.

More and more online merchants are cropping up all the time, so keep your eye out for new outlets. Some of the best and most comprehensive include www.glutenfreemall.com, www.gluten-free.net, www.amazon.com (look in the grocery, gluten-free section), www.glutensolutions.com, and www.glutenfree.com. Many Web sites allow you to learn more about products, recipes, and merchants and purchase a variety of products that can be shipped directly to you.

If there is a store nearby that carries many gluten-free options, try to browse their aisles first, before being overwhelmed by online options. Check to see if they ever have gluten-free sampling days or if distributors or manufacturers ever come by for in-store events. It is also good to form a relationship with these stores, as they will order products for you if they have a distributor and they are often a good resource for information on gluten-free cooking classes, support groups, and other activities.

Another option altogether is shopping at Asian groceries. Opinion is mixed in the celiac community as to whether these stores offer uncontaminated foods, since there is currently no certification procedure in place at these overseas plants. You will need to judge and decide for yourself, but there are far more gluten-free grains produced and milled in Asia on the whole than in Western regions, as gluten-free grains such as rice are still their staples. You will find in a cursory review of these grocers' aisles that they offer many gluten-free flours in larger packages for far cheaper prices than do Western-style grocers.

6. GATHER RESOURCES TO TAKE WITH YOU WHILE YOU SHOP

Copy, print out, or purchase lists of allowable and forbidden ingredients (you can even make a copy of lists from this book) and take the lists with you on your first few shopping trips. Ordinary grocery stores are where you will find these resources most useful, as many products available in those stores are gluten-free but are not necessarily marketed as gluten-free. Federal food labeling laws have helped, but it is comforting to have the lists for reference in case you encounter unusual ingredients.

Look for special gluten-free or natural food sections of supermarkets for foods and ingredients the stores may have not integrated into their regular food aisles. More and more major grocery chains are integrating such foods throughout the store, however, so it will be useful to take a complete tour of

Gluten-Free Living Consultants

If these tasks still seem overwhelming, if you are dealing with other food re-strictions besides celiac disease (or have a particularly picky child!), or if you feel that you need to learn how to live gluten-free yesterday, then hiring a con-sultant may be the smart thing to do. A consultant trained in gluten-free cook-ing and living can help you clean out your pantry, formulate a shopping list, devise recipes specific to your family's needs and tastes, and go shopping with you for your first comprehensive trip. For many, this option gets you on the road to living "normally" gluten-free much faster and actually saves you so much money in the long run, since you will really only be buying what you need and what brands actually taste good, rather than impulse buys that are later tossed because they tasted like the cardboard they were packaged in. I have spoken with too many mothers who have stood alone in the shopping aisles and cried about the overwhelming task of finding gluten-free foods their chil-dren (and/or the rest of their family) would actually eat, to underestimate the value of a skilled aid early in this process.

Evaluate your own needs, the resources available to you, and the amount of sleep you are losing over this integration to determine if you should look to someone to help you or if you are eager for the challenge on your own. Learn-ing how to shop gluten-free is absolutely doable, but your individual circum-stances may make it practical to briefly hire a professional to help you get back on the road to eating and living well.

the stores where you shop most frequently, simply to find where gluten-free items are likely to be kept, and also to compare prices from store to store.

Organic markets and health food stores cater to the needs of consumers with special diet requests such as gluten-free. Obviously, shopping in these aisles is far easier, but you will quickly find that it is far more expensive as well.[4] Many of these products are worth the price, and it may be worth the peace of mind in the beginning for you to stick only to brands clearly labeled

---

4. Pam Cureton, "The Gluten-Free Diet: Can Your Patient Afford It?" *Practical Gastroenterologist* (April 2007): 75–84, The Celiac Diet, Series #8, Carol Rees Parrish, ed.

gluten-free. However, there is simply no good reason for you to have to purchase your pasta sauce or ready-made frosting at a premium from a specially designated gluten-free vendor unless you just prefer the taste or particular ingredients of those brands. Armed with your gluten-free ingredient lists, you can feel confident purchasing some food items for your family at stores where the cost is not so great; save the expensive purchases for those which are necessarily made at specialty stores from specialty brands.

I realize that some might take issue with this recommendation, but having lived gluten-free for nearly ten years myself, I have had to learn to budget my food resources wisely. I share this piece of advice with you so that you may benefit from my hard-earned experience! Save your pennies for the gluten-free nutrition bars, pretzels, bagels, flour, mixes, pasta, and other items that are not available from ordinary manufacturers in ordinary supermarkets. Over time, more and more of these specially designated gluten-free items will be available from your local grocer and we can all look forward to easier and cheaper shopping trips! Until then, be smart about your purchases and you will have a happier tummy and wallet!

Shopping Gluten-Free in Six Easy Steps

1. Choose an all-purpose gluten-free flour mixture or recipe.
2. Pick your favorite snacks.
3. Identify meal ingredients.
4. Add some cooking essentials.
5. Choose your shopping venue.
6. Gather resources to take with you while you shop.

IN A SENTENCE

Finding a good gluten-free all-purpose flour mixture, having safe snacks, identifying meal menus that can be modified minimally, and figuring out where and how to shop will set you up for success and make food preparation much less daunting.

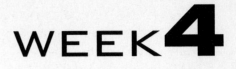

WEEK 4

learning

Seeking Support

WHEN I was diagnosed with celiac disease, I lived in a relatively rural area in the Midwest and I knew no one else who had ever heard of, much less shared in, celiac disease. Had there been an opportunity for me to interact with anyone else who ate gluten-free, that poor soul probably would have had to relocate or at least to block my persistent calls at some point. Upon a life-changing diagnosis like CD, most people feel lost. There are simply too many questions, too many contradictory opinions, too much opportunity for cross-contamination and confusion, and too many conflicting emotions to sort through successfully alone. Granted, I made it on my own, but it took me years to find an equilibrium, not to mention countless days of depression, grief, and self-pity before I could see the ultimate value in my diagnosis.

A lot of time has passed since that lonely time, and folks a lot smarter than I am have fortunately devised a wonderful solution to this problem of ignorance and isolation. Around the country and around the world, celiacs have begun to band together to share recipes, restaurant recommendations, support, and social normalcy. Some might view these organizations as a kind of 12-step program that graduates celiacs when they learn how to live gluten-free; others might stereotype the organizations as superficial social clubs with merely an unusual membership qualification. Neither is true. Instead, these groups are comprised of people who join and who stay, enjoying both the camaraderie and the constant influx of new approaches to living a better gluten-free life.

I recommend looking for a local celiac support group to anyone young or old who is newly diagnosed. Even many seasoned celiac veterans find that they gain invaluable information and friendship when they move or experience other life changes, such as having children. Newer groups started specifically for celiac parents and children (Cel-Kids and Raising Our Celiac Kids, a.k.a. ROCK) have been exceedingly popular and are spreading. Should you find yourself in an area without an established group, nothing should hold you back from starting your own! Your gastroenterologist or local dietitian is a great place to start for information, and the many lists available on the Internet will help you locate others nearby who would love to join you. Otherwise, Internet forums maintained on such sites as www.yahoo.com,[1] as well as celiac Listservs[2], offer a virtual support group environment and a 24-hour hotline to other celiacs around the world. One of the best is literally named the "Celiac Listserv" and boasts at least thirty-four hundred fellow celiac members from over thirty-three countries. This Listserv is an open, unmoderated discussion maintained via e-mail broadcasts to its members. Subscriptions are free and offer automatically e-mailed questions and answers in your inbox as often as you choose to receive them. Subscribe at celiac-subscribe-request@listserv.icors.org.

I never saw myself as the "support group" type, but I've come to recognize the value of finding a celiac family, particularly for the newly diagnosed. It is as equally rewarding to be on the receiving end of gluten-free information from fellow celiacs as it is to be able to hold the hands of those who are new to this disease and show them the shortcuts to a fulfilling gluten-free life. I am now proud to be a member of a celiac support group, myself, and when I travel to speak at other celiac support groups around the country, I enthusiastically share my knowledge with them.

---

1. Go to http://health.dir.groups.yahoo.com/dir/Health_Wellness/Support/Diseases_and_Conditions/ Celiac_Disease?st=10 for a list of groups maintained in various geographic regions.

2. A "Listserv" is a relatively new term in Internet lingo. Members of a Listserve are able to e-mail the entire list of members at one stroke: each e-mail message is automatically broadcast to the list and only members of the list may view the contents of these e-mail communications.

Support in Times of Trial and Temptation

I have heard too many stories to disregard the value of support groups. Members of celiac support groups have changed the lives of those who feel overwhelmed by their diagnosis, and aided families that are in crisis because a child is resisting compliance with the diet. People cannot fully understand the challenges that face you or your children unless they have walked in your shoes—these groups have worn those shoes and can provide not only information but ideas of how to overcome temptation or to successfully speak to a celiac family member about his or her new lifestyle.

Depending on how long you have been living gluten-free, you may feel more or less tempted to cheat on the dietary recommendations. The more you internalize and truly own the diagnosis, the less likely you will eat foods that contain gluten. Now that you understand how harmful gluten can be to a celiac body, you should not take this issue lightly. Depending on how sick you were and for how long before you were accurately diagnosed, the thought of cheating may be the farthest thing from your mind. However, particularly for parents of young celiacs, the gluten-free path can seem to be a long road fraught with glutenous potholes.

Children diagnosed with celiac disease face unique burdens as they grow up and mature. Pizza parties, birthday cakes, and "normal" eating at social events become really big deals when kids hit adolescence. Many celiac adolescents begin to resent not only the disease but the parents whom they may see as making them stand out by enforcing a different diet. Kids at every age crave control, and food restrictions take control away from them. It is easy to see why they would resist compliance with both the diet and the enforcer. Teenagers especially also think they are immortal, and they often simultaneously begin to think their parents are out of touch and wrong most of the time. The combination can be disastrous for a teen who makes the decision to eat gluten despite his or her parents' cautionary words.[3]

Recent research has yielded surprising and unsettling findings on adolescents who were diagnosed with celiac disease during childhood. Although compliance with a gluten-free diet led to remission of the disease in these

---

3. L. Greco et al., "'Compliance to a Gluten-Free Diet in Adolescents,' or 'What Do 300 Cœliac Adolescents Eat Every Day?'" *Italian Journal of Gastroenterology and Hepatology* 29, no. 4 (August 1997): 305–10.

children, statistics demonstrated a threefold higher mortality rate in these adolescents than in a celiac population diagnosed in adulthood. This mortality increase was largely due to suicide, accidents, and violence; however, researchers speculate that a high proportion of teenage noncompliance with a gluten-free diet was actually to blame.[4]

The isolation, embarrassment, and frustration that correspond with being different, particularly in the twelve- to seventeen-year-old celiac population, can lead to depression and anger, which can drive these kids to noncompliance or worse. Resulting gluten exposure can then cause actual changes in brain chemistry, which may lead to more aggressive, depressive behavior.[5] Many adult and adolescent celiacs describe a brain fog and an inability to concentrate when they have eaten gluten. Combine this with documented personality changes sometimes seen in other celiacs who are not gluten-free, and the results of noncompliance in a child or adolescent may be disastrous. Even if the child does not become violent or aggressive, it is difficult to imagine how depression would not take hold if he or she could no longer concentrate in school, was doing poorly in classes or other activities, and was suffering socially.[6] These issues were the subject of over twenty published e-mails exchanged between members of the international celiac Listserv

---

4. Kate Johnson, "Unexpected Health Risks Found in Celiac Patients," Entrepreneur.com (November 2007), http://www.entrepreneur.com/tradejournals/article/172316606_1.html (quoting Dr. Stephano Guandalini, chief of pediatric gastroenterology and director of the Celiac Disease Program at the University of Chicago, as well as Jessica Edwards George, PhD, psychologist and researcher at the Celiac Center at Beth Israel Deaconess Medical Center in Boston).

5. Kate, Johnson, "Unexpected Health Risks Found in Celiac Patients," Entrepreneur.com (November 2007), http://www.entrepreneur.com/tradejournals/article/172316606_1.html (quoting Dr. Stephano Guandalini, chief of pediatric gastroenterology and director of the Celiac Disease Program at the University of Chicago, "I am personally convinced that eating gluten if you have celiac disease really induced serious changes in brain chemistry that would make you inclined to aggressive, depressive behavior and therefore expose you to this risk."); Scot Lewey, "Brain and Neurological Problems Affect Almost Half of Celiacs Even with a Gluten-Free Diet," http://ezinearticles.com/?Brain-and-Neurological-Problems-Affect-Almost-Half-of-Celiacs-Even-with-a-Gluten-Free-Diet&id=904155.

6. Much research has been dedicated to the connection between gluten and the neurological conditions of autism and ADHD. At least one recent study has found that as many as 33 percent of autistic children have gluten sensitivity, which at least exacerbates these neurological symptoms when the patients remain on a gluten-containing diet. Aristo Vojdani, "Long Distance Connection: Does Celiac Disease Make ADHD Worse?" *Bottom Line Daily Health News* (June 7, 2007) http://www.bottomlinesecrets.com/blpnet/article.html?article_id=34378.

recently, demonstrating both the pervasiveness of the problem and the ready access to support through these kinds of mediums.

The potentially profound effect of a gluten-free diet on the social lives of children and adolescents who are not yet developmentally capable of coping as adults should not be underestimated.[7] One mother at my most recent lecture on living gluten-free approached me afterward for ideas to help. Her eleven-year-old was already angry and defiant about sticking to the diet. She consistently vented her frustration by telling her mother, "I wish I was eighteen already, because then I could eat as much gluten as I wanted!" Parents are constantly challenged to find ways to protect their children's health and safety—adding celiac disease to that burden can at times feel simply overwhelming.

Make it a priority to maintain a relationship with your gastroenterologist. Regular celiac blood-testing in conjunction with these appointments is another way of monitoring the success your child is having on the diet. Use your gastroenterologist and any dietitians or other gluten-free experts at your disposal to work with your celiac children and convince them that the diet is not simply your way of making their life miserable! Let them shoulder a little of the blame. Involve other family members in enthusiastically sharing the gluten-free diet, to make the celiac children feel less singled out at mealtime. And reach out beyond your family: Celiac support groups for children and for parents of celiac children are the other crucial link to being effective in this important task. Having other celiac peers around, activities geared toward socializing normally despite CD, and opportunities to interact with other parents in similar situations can be absolutely invaluable.

Resisting temptation is sometimes hard enough to do by yourself and is always difficult when you are doing it on behalf of your children. It is essential to impress upon them at every age how important it is to keep their bodies healthy, to be able to achieve the things that *they* want to do: excel in sports, grow bigger, concentrate more easily and succeed in school, look attractive, and so on. Take advantage of all the resources at your disposal and never give up! The risk and the reward are too great.

---

7. Kate Johnson, "Unexpected Health Risks Found in Celiac Patients," Entrepreneur.com (November 2007), http://www.entrepreneur.com/tradejournals/article/172316606_1.html; Päivi A. Pynnönen et al., "Gluten-Free Diet May Alleviate Depressive and Behavioural Symptoms in Adolescents with Cœliac Disease: A Prospective Follow-Up Case-Series Study," *BMC Psychiatry* 5 (2005): 14.

Celiac Support Groups in the United States

See the appendix (page 249) for a list of support groups around the United States as a starting point in your search for a group near you. The sheer number of listed groups should inform you as to how many of your fellow celiacs believe in the value of these organizations. Periodically check this information against the regularly maintained listing on www.celiac.com to ensure you are accessing the most up-to-date information.

IN A SENTENCE

Children and adolescents with celiac disease face unique burdens in addition to the normal struggles of growing up, but no matter what your age, finding support from Listservs, Internet contacts, and face-to-face support groups can be valuable.

living

How Others Found Help . . . and You Can, Too

FINDING AN active support group in your area is not always as easy as checking the list provided in the appendix. Sometimes you need to take the initiative yourself to bond with others who are similarly situated and live nearby, or give direction to an existing group. Investing time and energy into starting or building a celiac support group can provide countless rewards to you and others in your community. Here, Pat shares her story of how to enhance the offerings of a local support group and thereby make it a large, thriving, and vibrant member-driven organization.

◇ ◇ ◇

Growing a Support Group: Patricia Minnigh's Story

I can't remember a time when I didn't have some kind of stomach problems. Looking back, I can see that I always had issues with constipation, unexplained stomach aches, acid reflux, low blood sugar, and many 24-hour stomach bugs. I now know that "silent" celiac disease has always been at the core of my health problems, but the active damage to my intestines was actually triggered by a traumatic bowel surgery in 2001, after which I couldn't seem to recover any energy.

If it hadn't been for a friend encouraging me to investigate celiac disease, I'm sure I would have been sick much longer. As it was, I spent the next one and a half years back and forth between doctors who had not even considered celiac disease as a possibility. After I inquired about testing for celiac disease and was finally diagnosed, I was told to go on a gluten-free diet and to seek out the help of a dietitian. *What in the world is gluten-free? What can I eat? What do I have to avoid?* The relief at having a diagnosis was overwhelmed by the mandatory change in my diet. I grew up in a good Texas home with plenty of bread and breaded, fried foods. Why me?

My doctor said that she thought there might be a local support group in the area, but she was unsure if it was still around. She gave me a name and phone number from her files to follow up on my own. I left her office in a bit of a trance.

The dietitian provided me with "can have" and "can't have" food lists, but the support group soon provided me the sense of community that only those who feel unique in today's society can understand.

It took an adjustment phase with celiac disease before I was ready to get really involved with the group. I had just turned my small business over to my daughter-in-law and felt I was ready to "get busy," so I contacted the two ladies who were running the support group to see if I could help in any way. They welcomed any help they could get, so the three of us formed the first steering committee for the Anne Arundel County Celiac Support Group.

The University of Maryland Center for Celiac Research gave us information on guest speakers who might benefit our group, and I started contacting some of these speakers. Sometimes they were available and we could afford them, and sometimes we couldn't. Our group of three would then meet and plan out our monthly support group meetings, which featured local and traveling speakers.

We initially met in a room in a medical office building, but I lobbied the Anne Arundel Medical Center's Sajak Pavilion Wellness Center to add us to their schedule of support groups that met there. After several months and the help of their two wonderful dietitians, we met there for the first time in July 2005. We were then put on the Wellness Center Support Group's Schedule for the second Friday of every month from 6:30 to 8:30 p.m. It was important to us to have monthly meetings at a set date and time so that members could count on those events.

Within the first year, we added four more people to the steering committee and our Web site www.celiacsonline.com was established. From the beginning, we chose to stay independent and, to date, we do not ask for dues. In 2006 we added a ROCK (Raising Our Celiac Kids) group to the mix and in 2007 we incorporated as the Chesapeake Celiac Support Group.

We have had fabulous presentations by Dr. Alessio Fasano (the director of the University of Maryland Center for Celiac Research [CFCR]); Pam Cureton (dietitian at CFCR); Shelley Case (cookbook author); Steven Plogsted (head pharmacist from the Columbus Children's Hospital); Dana Korn (cookbook author); Dr. Thomas O'Bryan and Jax Lowell (cookbook author); representatives from Triumph Dining and Executive Concepts; wonderful bakers such as Tenzo Artisan, Everybody Eats, and Grandma Whimsey's; online grocers Gluten-Free Pantry and Mrs. May's; and Jules Shepard (cookbook author).

We post fliers about our meetings at local food stores and in some doctor's offices, and our meetings are on the monthly schedule published by the Wellness Center. Our numbers have swelled from approximately 30 members (6 to 8 at every meeting) in 2005 to at least 150 members (25 to 30 at every meeting) today. We have a strong core group that has reached out to the community to host events such as "Gluten-Free Day" at local organic markets, where we educate people on celiac disease and shopping gluten-free, and an all-day Seminar/Food Fair with Dana Korn and Dr. Thomas O'Bryan.

I can't say enough about how important our support group has been to me. We have truly become an extended family. Being able to share experiences (both good and bad), successes (and mistakes), great gluten-free food, and educational resources is invaluable. I am proud to say that what I have learned over the past six years of being gluten-free has actually taught me to enjoy food more now than I ever did. I remember eating whatever was at hand (and too much of it) and not taking the time to taste or enjoy what I put in my mouth. Now, every month I get to taste and share recipes with the group and I look forward to learning more every day about gluten-free living.

I have moved miles away from the "Why me?" to "Why not me?"

◇ ◇ ◇

Even if you feel secure in your gluten-free world, a distant move can rock even the sturdiest boat. Finding a group in your new home can offer the peace of mind of quickly learning where to shop, where to dine, and with whom your children can easily socialize. Sarah shares her relief at finding such a group after her family moved across the country with Cody, her celiac toddler.

◇ ◇ ◇

Finding Help after a Move: Sarah and Cody's Story

Almost a year had gone by since my three-year-old was diagnosed with celiac disease, and we had gotten into a pretty good routine, when our lives took a turn. My husband accepted a new job a thousand miles away in Wisconsin. Now we were going to be in a place that we had never been and had no family around. My fears were not just about whether I could find gluten-free food locally, but would anybody up there understand? We got to our new house and then I found myself wondering how I would find what I needed for my son when I didn't even know how to get to a grocery store!

I called a pediatrician to set up appointments for my children and mentioned to the nurse that my son Cody had CD. She informed me that one of the doctors at the practice had family members with CD as well. I gave a big sigh of relief that our new doctor might actually understand! The doctor called me that afternoon to talk to me and give me information on two local support groups in the area.

I quickly called the local groups to see what kind of help they had to offer me for this major time of transition and I was amazed at the warm welcome we felt from them. If I had not had them to lean on, I don't know that our move would have gone so smoothly. They taught me so much about local resources, stores, and restaurants that were good at working with CD patrons. I was pleasantly surprised that people in our new hometown did understand what we were going through! I was even more surprised when I found that almost *all* the food I needed, I could get at the local grocery store only five miles from our house.

For our family it has been an amazing journey. We have had some difficult times, but we cherish that we have a happy and healthy three-year-old. For us, the most important part of living as a family with CD is mostly that— working and living as a family. We may not be able to live as spontaneously as we used to, because now we have to plan ahead so that we can account for food for Cody and where he can eat if we are out and about. We have learned to keep a box in the car packed with snacks in case something arrives that we have no control over. We have found that as difficult as living with CD can be from time to time, it has truly been a blessing for our family because it has brought us closer together and to our community. It is also amazing to me how experimenting in the kitchen with my children has become so enjoyable for all of us; now we truly enjoy our time cooking and eating together.

◇ ◇ ◇

IN A SENTENCE

The life change required with adopting a gluten-free lifestyle is not something that comes naturally to most of us—take advantage of the active and plentiful support groups available to ease the transition and help you feel less alone.

FIRST-MONTH MILESTONE

At the end of this first month, you can look back proudly on the amount of information you have taken in. Learning about celiac disease and the fundamentals of a gluten-free diet is quite an accomplishment. So far, we have learned:

○ WHAT IT MEANS TO HAVE CELIAC DISEASE

○ WHAT IT MEANS TO ADOPT A GLUTEN-FREE LIFESTYLE

○ THE FUNDAMENTALS OF CREATING A GLUTEN-FREE KITCHEN

○ HOW TO PREPARE FOR AND WHERE TO SHOP GLUTEN-FREE

○ WHY AND HOW TO UTILIZE LOCAL SUPPORT GROUPS

MONTH **2**

Sticky Situations

BY NOW we've certainly all found ourselves in sticky situations since our diagnoses. Maybe you had a lunch interview or a first date at a restaurant and were embarrassed about having to place a special order. Or maybe you were just faced with stressful temptations—like that bread basket on the table. Whatever the temptation you face, recognize that it won't be your last and that you must live with the consequences of your own actions. No one else at the table has to suffer from your choice to eat something your body thinks is toxic; thus, no one else should have any right to pressure or embarrass you into taking that step.

My consulting clients often describe a technique that has helped them to overcome these moments of weakness: They think of how many such challenges they have already survived and visualize these as achievements that they do not want to cheapen by cheating, even just once. It becomes a matter of pride at a certain point, in some ways not unlike the alcoholic who boasts that he hasn't had a drink in 357 days or the Atkins dieter who proudly displays how much too big her pants have become because she hasn't eaten a sandwich in six weeks. Of course, visualizing how sick you could become from cheating can also be a powerful deterrent. Whatever you do, never doubt that by eating gluten, you are harming yourself—whether you feel immediate physical repercussions from your actions or not.

You are still very new to living gluten-free and so can expect every experience to be new to you. Trust that by the end of this first year, you will be well on your way to creating your own central repository of explanations, excuses, and avoidance techniques to cope with all kinds of sticky situations. Before you know it, they won't be uncomfortable anymore.

I am often asked about dating with celiac disease. It seems to be a popular topic for discussion in my cooking classes, in particular, where a large group of all ages of men and women are gathered for the central purpose of learning new gluten-free cooking techniques, but where a core group of younger women invariably begins to groan about these types of sticky situations. For the first few dates, most people find that they do not want to raise the issue of CD. Having a disease—indeed, any kind of health condition—is not something you typically want someone to know about if they don't know much else about you. The fear is that the disease will become your defining feature and few people want that impression to be the one that lasts.

This same fear holds true for business lunches, interviews, meeting important people for the first time, and so on. It's perfectly fine to be open about your celiac condition up front. Yet understandably, many don't wish to focus on a perceived deficiency when they are trying to impress. The challenge in our food-centered social world then becomes how to enjoy a meal in these situations without the other party knowing about your dining disability. Once you get to know the other person better, you get the job or close the deal, you can inform and educate others about celiac in your new relationship in your own way. In the beginning, though, most seek ways to avoid having to engage in that conversation.

If this is you, there are several semisneaky ways to accomplish this goal, so never fear! One of the easiest is to control the location of the date or meeting. If you can choose where to go, you will already know the menu and be able to feel comfortable ordering without having to discuss anything unusual with the waiter or chef. Obviously, nicer restaurants do a better job of attending to individual eating preferences and restrictions, but you can even get by with many lower-priced Asian or Latin restaurants that offer many rice and corn dishes.

If you are unable to pick the restaurant but you know in advance where you are going, you can review the menu and ingredients online. I always suggest calling and speaking with the chef or manager before you go, if possible, as well, before even stepping foot inside the establishment. Contact the staff during their least busy hours—usually between two and four in the afternoon—and alert them to your needs while asking for advice on choosing a menu item. In conversation, you can also gain some confidence in their cross-contamination procedures and knowledge about food allergies and intolerances.

If you have no choice in the matter and no advance notice of the location, you still have options. Always carry a cook card with you (see Month 3)—you can discreetly slip it to the waiter when you step away to use the restroom before ordering. You can also take a side trip to the kitchen door and wait for a person of authority to intercept you so that you can have a full-blown discussion with them away from the table. If, for some reason, none of these tricks will work in your situation, scan the menu for something you consider to be a safe option by ordering it without sauces, toppings, and so on. Salads often fall into this category; if you ask for no croutons and for a dressing of just oil and vinegar, you are likely to have ordered well (remember, though, that if your salad comes with croutons on it, you must ask for another salad–don't just pick the croutons off, or you'll risk cross-contamination). Baked potatoes with steamed vegetables, or grilled seafood or chicken served over plain steamed brown or white rice without sauces are also fairly safe bets and do not draw unnecessary attention to your eating habits. For dessert, ice cream, sorbet, fresh fruit, and even crème brulée are usually celiac-friendly.

If you are unsure of yourself and would rather not order much food, you can claim to have eaten beforehand, or do the ever-popular, "I'm on a diet" routine. Feel out the situation and be resourceful—if there is simply no way you can find to feel comfortable over a meal during the early stages of dating, suggest meeting for coffee, going to the movies, or some other activity that does not center around food.

Otherwise, simply explain your dietary restrictions and do so in a positive light. Focus on all the benefits about your diagnosis, your current health, and the array of food options that remain available to you. If your date's eyes glaze over or he or she is otherwise unreceptive to your situation, then it is better that you didn't waste more time on that person anyway. The manner in which others handle your lifestyle and diagnosis is actually very telling. Consider yourself fortunate to have such a character test at your fingertips!

Tips for Gluten-Free Dating:

- ○ Pick the restaurant.
- ○ Review the menu and ingredients online in advance.
- ○ Call ahead and speak with the chef or manager.
- ○ Carry a Cook Card (see page 120).
- ○ Detour to the kitchen on the way to the bathroom to speak with the staff privately.
- ○ Order fresh and plain: something grilled or steamed without sauces.
- ○ Order a salad with oil and vinegar and no croutons.
- ○ Order fresh fruit, sorbet, or ice cream for dessert.
- ○ Suggest meeting somewhere that does not center around food.
- ○ Explain your food restrictions in a positive light.

Dining and Dating: Susie Delaney's Story

If you are single and you have celiac disease, then you have just hit the dating jackpot! I hear about the games my single friends play with people they are dating and I thank my lucky stars because I was given an automatic filter. Congratulations, celiacs, you have an instant barometer for judging how the person across the table feels about you. It all comes down to a simple question: how does your date treat your health/food restrictions?

If the man or woman you are with does his/her homework ahead of time, kudos to them, that person is worth another date. If when you order, you tell the server that you have a gluten/wheat allergy and the person you are with asks questions and engages you in conversation about it, the person is worth another date. Once your food arrives, if your date makes certain that what you've ordered is safe for you to eat, the person is worth another date. If your date also orders something gluten-free after learning about your restrictions, the person is worth another date. Are you starting to get the idea? If you pay attention, there are endless opportunities for your date to show you how much he or she is interested in you; celiac disease is to thank for all those opportunities.

Whether or not I'm on a date, I always identify myself to the waiter as gluten-free. My method is very simple and yields positive results 98 percent of the time. First and foremost, I learned early on that you get more with honey than you do with vinegar. It's not the waiter's responsibility to make sure you order properly to get a safe, delicious meal. Likewise, it's not your date's responsibility to make sure you're enjoying a gluten-free meal. Having said that, every waiter who does take your food restrictions seriously is worth a thank-you, and every date who goes the extra mile to ensure that you are enjoying a safe meal is worth another date.

The easiest way I've found to explain my restrictions to a server is to tell him or her that I'm allergic to wheat. I specify that I can't have flour, wheat, barley, or rye—for [the restaurant's] purposes, this means I can't have most grains. Considering my dietary restrictions, I first ask if there is anything that is easy for the chef to amend. Sometimes I stick to what the chef recommends; most often though, I choose the meal I want and the chef amends it to fit my diet. This approach yields a wonderful dining experience nearly every time: I walk away having educated a waiter about celiac disease; I enjoy a delicious meal; and I usually gain an appreciation for yet another person who took the time to make my health a priority.

I live in Washington, D.C., where fine dining options are endless. Even after being diagnosed with celiac disease, I still eat out on a regular basis. I started dating my Mr. Wonderful four months after I was diagnosed with celiac disease. There are many reasons why I ultimately fell in love with him, but his consideration for my diet and his genuine interest in my health was a major factor in the beginning. The value that he placed on my health from the beginning allowed me to see his generous and caring qualities very early in the relationship.

Having celiac disease has opened a world of doors to me. I experience and have appreciation for grains and foods that I never would have had an incentive to try if not for celiac disease. Every time a waiter listens enough to get it right, I am blessed. Every time a restaurant makes the extra effort to prepare a phenomenal gluten-free meal, they have won a lifelong customer. And most important, every time Mr. Wonderful goes out of his way to ensure that what I'm eating is safe, I fall in love with him a little more.

Having celiac and dating a new person is an exciting, unique opportunity to be with someone who genuinely loves you for who you are and who finds joy in the things that bring you happiness. So get out there! If you allow yourself, there's no doubt you'll meet your own wonderful person and enjoy a fabulous meal in the process.

◇ ◇ ◇

IN A SENTENCE

Don't be afraid to assert yourself, whether in front of your date or behind the scenes, to ensure you can go out again and enjoy yourself!

living

Overcoming College Challenges

OFTEN ONE of the hardest times in a person's life is the first year or two of college. On your own, often still in some form of teenage rebellion or experimental mode, and accountable to no one but yourself. These years can be even more difficult for young celiacs who are entering this uncharted territory and have no desire to draw attention to themselves as being "different." The best approach is often to take this seeming disadvantage and turn it into a way to meet people, help others, and effect change on campus. Many students have actually found their footing early because of having celiac disease. Two celiac college students now share their very different, yet equally challenging college experiences. These students both made positive things happen for themselves and for others, but on their own terms. The lessons learned from their positive attitudes and proactive approaches demonstrate inspiring results—which only occurred because they each had celiac disease!

◇ ◇ ◇

Fixing the Dining Hall: Chrissy Andrews's Story

Eating gluten-free with access to a health food store and your own kitchen is one thing. Eating gluten-free for the first time in a college dining hall that serves thousands of students daily is an entirely different experience. It was mid-January 2007, the beginning of my second semester in college, when I was first told that I "must have a strict and permanent gluten-free diet." It was impossible to understand the implications that this simple phrase would have on my life in even one year.

That first semester on a gluten-free diet was a struggle. I was a college student who could not drink beer, a Catholic who could not receive the Host, and an avid baker who could not eat anything containing flour. However, after spending a summer at home enjoying the support and help of my family, along with time, practice, and a lot of Internet research, I was soon on the path to a happy, healthy, gluten-free life.

I took my first step toward really normalizing my life at college by identifying the flaws and imperfections with my living situation. The dining hall setup was simply not good enough. Although a significant number of foods are naturally gluten-free (vegetables, eggs, meats, peanut butter, hummus), issues of cross-contamination in the buffet-style dining hall were of great concern to me.

Returning to school in the fall, I decided to help make a change so that eating could be safer and easier for me and the other students on campus who have to eat gluten-free (currently about fifteen other students, and increasing every year). After much brainstorming, I suggested creating a gluten-free room, complete with a full refrigerator and freezer stocked with gluten-free bread, lunch meat, soup, and prepared gluten-free food. In addition, the room would have a microwave, toaster, George Foreman grill, and waffle maker. All of the students requiring a gluten-free diet would have access to this room and the ability to prepare their meals to their own liking, supplementing their meal with other items from the regular dining hall as well. Campus food services supported the idea of a gluten-free room and, much to my delight, almost immediately started construction.

The room was finished before fall break and has made all the difference in my trips to the dining hall. The students who use this room trade their student ID for a key, enter the room, prepare their food, and then go into the dining hall with everyone else. The room is routinely stocked with items, including store-bought gluten-free cookies, crackers, chips, and bars that we are able to take from the room. Although the system is not perfect, it continues to improve and it has proven a success with the many students who use it.

To be able to see my idea turn into such a tangible reality is something that I have never achieved before and it is one of the things in my life that I feel most proud about accomplishing. Many people worked together to make the gluten-free room a reality and I hope that it will continue to improve people's lives long after I graduate.

I feel empowered by the fact that I feel I can be a normal college student, even with CD. I have never really felt that I have a disease per se, but that I just have some food restrictions that help me protect myself from future health issues. To be healthy without taking any medications is a real gift. Going off to college, I had an entire drawer full of medicine. Now, I only take a daily multivitamin. Having a food-related cure returned the power to me; whereas medicines have side effects and consequences associated with them, the food-related cure gave me the power over my own health.

There are so many ways in which I have benefited from my new gluten-free lifestyle. In the past year, I think I have seen more growth in myself than at any other time in my life. I have adjusted to having some attention on myself rather than blending into the background. I can better accept compliments for my accomplishments and am proud of the obstacles that I have overcome. I have grown closer to my family and realized how essential they are to me. I have discovered that my friends are always looking out for me.

In addition, my daily life has improved and become easier in a number of ways as well. I no longer have to make sure there are rest stops along the way if I want go for a run outside. I can eat less than two hours before bed without worrying whether my acid reflux will bother me all night. Best of all, I am really happy with my life and who I am, and although this is not just because I don't eat gluten, I would not trade anything to go back to a gluten-full world.

◇ ◇ ◇

Overcoming College Challenges while
Living Gluten-Free: Julianne Valle's Story

It will always be there: the temptation, the frustration, and the fading memories of crunchy toast in the morning. Trying to forget what my taste buds once enjoyed is nearly impossible, but accepting celiac and moving forward is something I accomplish every day. It took me a while to realize that celiac is something I should not be ashamed about, but rather an element in the mix of life that enhances my character.

I was nineteen and a freshman in college when I was diagnosed with celiac disease. I left my gastroenterologist's office that Wednesday morning with pictures of my insides, a photocopied sheet outlining what I could not eat, and substantial uncertainty. I had so many questions colliding in my head: *What does this mean? How much of my life am I going to have to change? Will I always have it? Why did I get this and why did I get it now? What's next?* This was the first time I had even heard of celiac and now I was officially diagnosed with this life-altering, taste-adjusting disease.

The reality of how much this disease was really going to affect my life did not sting me until a week later, when I visited a friend's house for the first time as a newly diagnosed celiac. It was a casual night, the ones young college friends have when you can wear a T-shirt and jeans and come late after your restaurant shift ends. Maintaining my shaky optimism became difficult when a beer was shoved in my hands after I walked through the front door. No one was paying attention to where the full cup of beer ended up, but I was overcome with uncertainty. Meanwhile, wafting in from the next room was the heavenly aroma of pizza that drove my senses into a weak frenzy.

I had always been a little shy, and now, trying to explain to a bunch of college kids why I could not indulge in the everyday simple things in life that, at that very moment, they were taking for granted was a lot harder than I had expected. The responses made me feel like I was different, not like them, and weird because I could not eat pizza or drink their cheap beer. I worried people thought I was a snob, or too good for their college lifestyle. It became tiring and redundant always explaining why I could not eat this or that. I did not want to have to incessantly give reasons for my seemingly odd behavior.

I had always thought college was fun and adventurous; I liked meeting new people and making new friends. What I had not envisioned was being ridiculed by my peers, being made fun of, and being called a cop-out for reasons they never even wanted to understand. So I distanced myself from making new friends or showing up at a college party; instead, I asked for more hours at work to take up any free time and spent the other nights at home studying where I could thrive inside a comfort zone of acceptance and compassion for my differences. Even though my sister made me inedible garlic bread, my dad brought me homemade cookies that tasted like sawdust, and my brother always said, "At least it's not me," this was the place where judgment was left at the door and tears of frustration were always comforted.

After living at home with celiac for a year and a half while attending a community college, I transferred to the University of Maryland–College Park to complete my undergraduate degree. For the first time I was going to be living away from home, away from the ease of knowing everyone around me "got" it, and embarking yet again on a quest of acceptance from my peers. I realized that I would have to step up and face all the things that knocked me down before.

I moved into a house off-campus with five other young ladies. On the day I moved in, my mom brought her big fat permanent marker to label all my food, my own jar of jelly, and her homemade gluten-free dinners wrapped in aluminum foil with "GF" written in enormous letters. Not only was I a little terrified, but so was my mom. This was a new start for me and, with it, I promised myself that celiac disease would no longer have control over my life; I would be the one in power now.

What scared me the most about moving into a house with total strangers was revealing all of my diet restrictions and explaining that every one of my roommates was going to be affected by them on some level. I spent a lot of time devising how I was going to explain my condition, as I didn't think that announcing that I had celiac disease would make a good first impression. Yet they obviously had to know about it if I was to share a house and, more important, a kitchen with them. I had to make sure I covered all the basics: cross-contamination, having my own condiments, and not to "help" themselves to my gluten-free food.

While I was considering how to break this news to them, one of my new roommates poked her head in my bedroom and asked, "Do you have celiac?" I was completely caught off-guard but felt a huge smile stretch across my face as a sensation of reassurance filled the void I dreaded would exist between me and my new roommates. Virginia did not have the disease herself but had heard about it and, to my surprise, knew a lot about CD.

It is two years later and I still live with Virginia and she has become a vital support system for me, especially in social settings with a young crowd. During those college games of beer pong, Virginia is the one who drinks wine with me instead of beer. It is securing to know that my friends will go above and beyond to make sure my accommodations are considered.

There were many times I was extremely envious of what my roommates were eating, but at the same time, I know they were all very jealous of the special baked brownies and cookies my mom always sent me. I have been lucky that they were receptive to learning about celiac and understood the importance of avoiding cross-contamination in our kitchen. While I know they tried to be conscious of my needs, I still kept disinfectant wipes close on hand, which I used to wash off the countertops before I cooked something, and rewashed the pans and pots I would use to cook with as well. It was nearly impossible to share food, but there were times when we did all sit down to eat dinner together for special occasions when we made everything gluten-free. It makes me feel special when meals are prepared around me and at the same time is a significant learning experience for everyone involved. For my birthday, my roommates even made an exclusive trip to the organic market to buy gluten-free cake mix.

Today, I cannot begin to imagine life without having celiac disease. I cannot deny that it might be a little more convenient, but at the same time, I would lose the exploration and persistence that flourishes within this challenging lifestyle. Celiac disease is something I never asked for, but I now know that it has not thrown me off course, rather it put me on a better path.

◇ ◇ ◇

IN A SENTENCE

> *College life can be both a challenge and an opportunity for those with celiac disease who approach it with resourceful optimism.*

learning

Can You Drink Alcohol?

BY NOW you understand that wheat, barley, and rye—and any derivatives thereof—are strictly forbidden on a gluten-free diet. You have had months of learning and living by these rules, so what I am going to tell you now might not make sense at first blush: you can enjoy distilled alcoholic drinks even if they are made from wheat, barley, or rye! The key here is "distilled." The distillation process, during which carbohydrate-containing plants ferment and produce alcoholic liquids, which are then chemically separated, effectively weeds out larger particles like gluten peptides, rendering the remaining liquid gluten-free.

This revelation is a relatively recent one. When I was diagnosed with CD in 1999, there was something of a controversy over what alcoholic beverages were gluten-free, with wine and certain liquors such as tequila and light rum being the only ones on which everyone could agree as being gluten-free. In fact, the first publication of my cookbook, *Nearly Normal Cooking for Gluten-Free Eating*, listed those alcohols as the only assuredly safe ones for celiacs. Things move fast in the world of gluten-free food and drink: my book and conventional wisdom have

Popular Gluten-Free Brews Available in the U.S.

Bard's Tale—www.bardsbeer.com

New Grist—www.lakefrontbrewery.com/sorghum.html

Green's—www.glutenfreebeers.co.uk/; distributed in the United States by Merchant du Vin—www.merchantduvin.com/pages/5_breweries/greens.html:

    Green's Discovery—Amber Ale

    Green's Endeavour—Dubbel Dark Ale

    Green's Explorer—Quest Triple Blonde Ale

Hambleton Ales—http://www.hambletonales.co.uk/gfa.htm:

    GFA Pale Ale

    GFL Pale Lager

Ramapo Valley Brewery Honey Beer—
www.rvbrewery.com/html/honey_beer.html

Gluten-Free Alcoholic Beverages

For ease of reference, I have listed below some of the most popular alcohols that are gluten-free:

Armagnac	Grappa	Scotch whiskey
Bailey's Irish Cream	Jägermeister	Sherry
Brandy	Kahlúa	Tequila
Bourbon	Mead	Vermouth
Champagne	Ouzo	Vodka
Cider (as long as there are no barley additives)	Rum	Whiskey
Cognac	Sake (unless rice syrup or other barley additives are included)	Wine (including ports, sherries, and sparkling wine)
Frangelico		
Gin		

now espoused the nearly universally accepted principle that "[d]istilled products do not contain any harmful gluten peptides."[1]

The acceptable alcohol list does have its limits though, and it is important to remember the distillation rule: *Other alcohols that are grain-based and not*

---

1. Healthlink, "Celiac Disease," Medical College of Wisconsin, http://healthlink.mcw.edu/article/956622658.html.

distilled, such as malt beverages like many wine coolers and most beers, are ab-solutely not *safe for those on a gluten-free diet.*

As for beer, it has come a long way as well. Just a few short years ago, there was no such thing as a commercially available gluten-free beer. Thankfully, though, nationally and internationally distributed gluten-free beers are now available that do a mighty tasty job of filling the beer void for celiacs. These manufacturers are using such ingredients as sorghum and millet to produce gluten-free alternatives we can now enjoy. One with the widest distribution in the United States is Redbridge Beer made by Anheuser-Busch. Nearly all restaurants, bars, and alcohol sales outlets have distributors that carry An-heuser-Busch products. Thus, if you are interested in trying this brew, simply ask your favorite establishment to request it on their next shipment. It comes in draft and bottle. For more information on this sorghum-based lager, go to www.redbridgebeer.com/about/aboutRedbridge.aspx.

Some other interesting Web sites are fun to check for the latest listing of companies that declare their drinks gluten-free. One that seems to be up-dated regularly is www.glutenfreedrinks.com; www.celiac.com also posts arti-cles on any new developments in the gluten-free marketplace. In addition to these listings of gluten-free alcohols, check for information on cocktail mixes as well. Many mixed drinks such as margarita, martini, Tom Collins, and Bloody Mary are gluten-free. As with any other gluten-free food item, though, you should read labels closely for these drinks if they are being made from a mix, since some manufacturers add non-gluten-free flavorings and additives.

Want to raise a toast to your new, gluten-free lifestyle? As you can see, we celiacs have many libations at our disposal, including some made with wheat, barley, and rye that are rendered safe through the distillation process. Even major commercial beer breweries are getting in on the act, expanding still further the choices we can raise in that toast.

IN A SENTENCE

The distillation process removes gluten peptides from many popular alco-holic drinks, which, when combined with the growing list of gluten-free beers and a long list of always safe drinks, gives celiacs an ever-lengthening list of beverages from which to choose.

living

Dining Out
Again—Safely and Enjoyably

WHEN ASKED if I eat out at restaurants now that I have celiac disease, I always reply with a resounding, "YES!" I routinely encourage my consulting clients to go out to eat and enjoy restaurants again, as well. Now, I always follow that up with lots of advice on how to do so intelligently and safely, so I will do the same here.

Before you were diagnosed with celiac disease, running out to grab a quick bite to eat where someone else had to do the cooking and cleaning up was a luxury you may not have fully appreciated. Now that you have some idea of the hazards of eating gluten, you may feel too frightened to leave the confines of your own (now) gluten-free kitchen. A recent study of Canadians living with CD reported that more than half of the families with celiac members reported that they avoided restaurants all or most of the time,[2] despite the fact that four out of five people

---

2. M. Rashid et al., "Celiac Disease: Evaluation of the Diagnosis and Dietary Compliance in Canadian Children," *Pediatrics* 116, no. 6 (2005): 754–59.

generally report that going out to eat at a restaurant is a better way to use their leisure time than cooking and cleaning up![3]

Living gluten-free is not about living in a bubble, though, so I urge you to put your fears on the shelf of your gluten-free flour cupboard and close the door! Since 49 percent of celiacs apparently believe that their quality of life would be improved if there were more gluten-free choices at restaurants, it is imperative that you learn how to successfully navigate the restaurant world as a celiac wanting to live a better life. There is a way to safely go back out again and socialize, entertain, "do business lunches," go on dinner dates, and grab a meal at a local joint. You just have to know how to do it!

Before you run back out to McDonald's, a few important pointers are useful:

1. Try to eat early or late so that you are avoiding the rush hours when the managers and chefs have the least time to pay special attention to your meal. Also, wherever possible, dine at restaurants that make their food from scratch. I know it's not always easy to do, and I know that those restaurants are likely to be more expensive, but they will have a much better grip on what their ingredients are. Besides, aren't you worth it? Your health certainly is!

2. Understand the limitations of larger restaurants and fast-food chains. They work with premade sauces and ingredients, have line cooks preparing different parts of the same meal, usually have unseasoned staff (pun intended), and cross-contamination is often hard to avoid. Check such resources as the national Gluten Intolerance Group (GIG), which maintain free lists of restaurants participating in the Gluten-Free Restaurant Awareness Program (www.glutenfreerestaurants.org/) or go to www.clanthompson.com/celiacstore/, which sells pocket guides to gluten-free restaurants, foods, prescriptions, over-the-counter drugs, and beer, wine, and spirits. No matter what the size of the restaurant, be sure to patronize restaurants on these lists wherever possible, to encourage them to continue gluten-free offerings, and to relieve your own mind about your meal.

3. When possible, call ahead during less busy times and ask questions about the menu and alert the chef of your needs. When you arrive at the restaurant, use "cook cards" (see text box) to minimize misunderstandings between you and the kitchen. Waiters love these cards because they don't have to write all of your ingredient restrictions down and they are absolved

---

3. National Restaurant Association, "2008 Restaurant Industry Facts," www.restaurant.org/research/ind_glance.cfm.

of responsibility when they can hand the cards to the kitchen. The kitchen staff appreciates the cards because they are not left in the dark as to the parameters of your food restrictions. And you'll love the cards because they make your life a lot easier and safer. As long as there is good communication between you and the kitchen, you should feel more comfortable with your entire dining experience. Also be sure to tip your server well—it never hurts to reward and give incentive to servers for your next visit!

Cook Card

I Cannot Eat (gluten, wheat . . .) _____!

I am allergic or intolerant of _____ *and any related ingredients. Some examples of products containing this food include:*

√ *Please substitute any ingredients which may contain these types of foods with other safe food choices that you would recommend.*
√ *Please prepare my food away from any dishes containing these prohibited ingredients.*
√ *Please clean any surfaces which may have become contaminated with these prohibited ingredients.*
√ *Please wash any utensils and pans which may have become contaminated with these prohibited ingredients.*

Thank you so much for helping me to safely enjoy your wonderful food!

Copyright Jules E. D. Shepard, Nearly Normal Cooking, LLC 2008

4. Establish a relationship with the manager or owner of a few restaurants you particularly enjoy. Maybe it's the neighborhood Italian restaurant or a take-out Chinese place you have always loved, or even a chain restaurant that is close to work and your colleagues love to frequent. Introduce yourself sometime and educate the proprietor about your food restrictions in the kindest possible way. Offer to go over the menu items with him or her (during off-peak hours!) and to identify what is already gluten-free so that they can let other patrons know about safe choices. Ask if you could make arrangements to bring your own gluten-free pasta and have the chef boil it for you in a separate pot but serve his recommended (gluten-free) sauces. Volunteer to let the local celiac support group know of this restaurant's cooperation and drum up support for the establishment. Get creative and, by all means, be nice! You may even be surprised at how eager they are to please you when you become a regular and are greeted at the door like Norm on *Cheers*.

5. Double-check about the fryer. It is easy to believe that the fries you are ordering are gluten-free because potatoes are on your safe list. However, restaurants often have only one fryer, and once your french fries have been deep-fried in the oil they also used to fry the chicken nuggets, your fries are no longer gluten-free. Furthermore, even if their fryer is not cross-contaminated from other food items, the french fries may themselves *not* be gluten-free! McDonald's famous french fries are a perfect example. Their Web site has from time to time indicated that their fries are free from wheat and gluten; however, numerous lawsuits (another suit is pending in Texas as of February 2008) have alleged that the food allergy listing on the site is incorrect and misleading. Due to these lawsuits, the Web site now indicates that the vegetable oil in which the fries are cooked actually contains beef flavor derived from wheat and milk![4] Thus, seemingly gluten-free items (potatoes + vegetable oil) may still contain gluten—it never hurts to check.

6. While you're at it, ask that your food be prepared on aluminum foil. Whether you order a grilled steak or a sautéed fish, ask that the chef place foil under your food. This request does three things in addition to actually protecting against cross-contamination. First, it brings attention to the fact that gluten-containing food may have been on that grill first. Second, it causes the cook to actually stop to consider whether he or she is using a clean pan to flash-fry your fillet. Third, it ensures that the kitchen will take your food restriction much more seriously.

6. Avoid cafeterias. Not that I harbor any childhood resentment from being forced to eat lime Jell-O, succotash, corn pudding, fried catfish, and a yeast roll (all on the same plate), but you get my point. It doesn't matter here if the kitchen can somehow avoid cross-contamination; the line probably can't. The same serving spoon that was in that corn pudding will likely find its way into your steamed vegetables at some point. It's a sad truth, but no less truthful.

7. Thank all those at the restaurant who were helpful and attentive, and be sure to leave a generous tip. This gratitude will come back in spades, at this and other restaurants, for you and for other diners with food restrictions.

Every day, it seems, another restaurant produces a gluten-free menu, so stay tuned to the celiac network to learn of new options. Bonefish Grill,

---

4. Http://app.mcdonalds.com/bagamcmeal?process=item&itemID=6050; the Celiac Sprue Association released a "February 2006 Statement on McDonald's French Fries," which indicated that these products "might be considered, commercially, to 'contain no gluten,'" as several factors reduced the initial level of gluten from the original wheat-based flavoring ingredient. The document also recommended that celiacs make their own personal diet choices after gathering all of the information. http://www.csaceliacs.org/documents/FinalCSAStatementMcDonalds023006wlh.pdf.

Carrabba's Italian Grill, Legal Seafood, Outback Steakhouse, and P. F. Chang's China Bistro have all proven among the nicer chain restaurants that maintaining gluten-free options is not only possible, but profitable. Following their lead, we can look forward to many more restaurants breaking into this market in the future. Until then, though, follow the tips I have listed for you above, and be sure to let all the restaurants you visit know that you are eating gluten-free and would love to see more options. The bottom line is that consumer demand drives results, so don't be shy!

Fast-Food Fare

Although I would never recommend that someone on a gluten-free diet frequent fast-food restaurants, I also live in the same world you do. I recognize that sometimes there are not a lot of choices and planning ahead is not a luxury you always have. So, with that in mind and with the added caveat that I am not endorsing any of these restaurants (nor am I intentionally excluding any other fast-food restaurants), I have compiled a partial list of national chain restaurants that you may wish to check out.

To explain, I researched a host of different chain restaurants and included only those with specific food allergy Web pages that showed at least some gluten-free options (and thereby demonstrated some understanding of gluten). Granted, corn-on-the cob and coleslaw might not be your idea of adequate options, but if you are expecting to grab a gluten-free meal at KFC, then you've already got a problem! In all seriousness, though, some of these restaurants have done a nice job of laying out several gluten-free options that you might want to print out in case of emergency. I recommend keeping this list in your glove compartment right next to a couple of gluten-free snack bars (such as Larabars), so you do actually have options.

I have not provided the exact menu items for each restaurant, although to generalize, many milk shakes and ice creams are gluten-free (provided you don't get toppings or cones); also, sandwiches served without bun, and salads without croutons and served with oil and vinegar, are more likely to be gluten-free. However, as you have learned over the past two months of living gluten-free, you must always double-check ingredients! Just as food manufacturers change their ingredients from time to time, so, too, do restaurants. Do your homework, check the current listings, and go through that drive-through armed with the information you need to place an educated order.

Some Celiac-Friendly Fast-Food Options

A&W	www.awrestaurants.com/nutrition/default.htm
Arby's	www.arbys.com/nutrition/printable.php?type=allergens
Baskin-Robbins	www.baskinrobbins.com/Nutrition/allergen.aspx
Blimpie	www.blimpie.com/na/index.php
Burger King	www.bk.com/Nutrition/PDFs/ingredients.pdf
Carvel	www.carvel.com/faq/faq.htm#ng
Chick-Fil-A	www.chick-fil-a.com/#gluten
Chipotle	www.chipotle.com/#flash/food_ingredients
Chuck E. Cheese's	www.chuckecheese.com/menu/allergy-information.php
Dairy Queen	www.dairyqueen.com/us-en/eats-and-treats/gluten-free-products/
Hardee's	www.hardees.com/content/downloads/ingredients_allergens.pdf
Jack-in-the-Box	www.jackinthebox.com/ourfood/ingredients.php
KFC	www.yum.com/nutrition/allergen/allergen_kfc.asp
Long John Silver's	www.yum.com/nutrition/allergen/allergen_ljs.asp
McDonald's	www.mcdonalds.com/app_controller.nutrition.categories.ingredients.index.html
Pei Wei	www.peiwei.com/glutenfreeMenu.htm
Pizza Hut	www.yum.com/nutrition/allergen/allergen_ph.asp
Subway	www.subway.com/subwayroot/MenuNutrition/Nutrition/pdf/AllergenChart.pdf
Taco Bell	www.yum.com/nutrition/documents/tb_ingredient_statement.pdf
Taco del Mar	www.tacodelmar.com/food/gluten.html
Wendy's	www.wendys.com/food/Nutrition.jsp

IN A SENTENCE

You don't have to give up on dining out—you can work with restaurant personnel before and during meals, and you may even enjoy safe fast-food experiences when you know what to look for and consciously avoid cross-contamination.

MONTH **4**

learning

Talking with Friends about Celiac Disease

NOW THAT you are beginning to fully grasp the implications of celiac disease, recognize the symptoms that were overlooked by the medical community in your own or in others' misdiagnoses, and see the possibilities for future health and happiness while following a gluten-free diet, it is hard not to begin to "diagnose" everyone around you with this condition. Knowing the sheer number of possible symptoms by which the disease can mask itself, and simultaneously understanding how truly common it is, I sometimes feel compelled to encourage others to get tested, if only to rule out the possibility of CD. It is a strange irony—a remarkably common disease that most know little about.

Intellectually, it makes sense that physicians treating folks with any kind of otherwise undiagnosed or unresolved health condition should include celiac in their battery of other serological testing. If they are going to order lab tests anyway, why not add the celiac panel to their other tests? These blood tests are now common, quite accurate, and covered by most insurance.

Until recently, in Italy, *every child* was screened for CD by age six, so this concept couldn't be that outrageous![1]

I always have to caution myself that another individual's health is a very personal matter. But I do try to educate people about CD as often as possible; let them internalize the information and use it as they will. Perhaps it will resonate with them and be the impetus they need to inquire about it with their physician. Or maybe my descriptions of symptoms sound familiar to them in someone they know and love, and they will in turn inform those people of their need for testing.

In advance of a book signing I was doing near my parents' home town, my mother was discussing with her hairdresser that I was coming for the event. Her hairdresser was curious as to what gluten and celiac disease were, exactly, and as my mother described the disease, her hairdresser's face grew more and more concerned. Finally, she put her scissors down and excused herself to make a personal call. She telephoned her best friend and said, "I think you have celiac disease." Her friend had also never heard of CD but, upon hearing this information, began researching it on the Internet. By the time she came in the next morning to meet me at my book signing, she, her father, and her uncles were all convinced that they had celiac disease.

This young woman—barely younger than I—was the first person at my signing. She and her father were eagerly awaiting my arrival and bombarded me with questions. Apparently, her whole father's side of the family just thought they had "bad guts": near constant bloating, diarrhea, gas, and weight gain affected her father and all of his brothers. The young woman was very attractive but was wearing oversized clothes that hid her body shape and size.

In the course of our discussion, she confided to me that these types of elastic-waist clothes were the only things she could wear anymore, because she never knew from one day to the next what size pants she could fit into. Bloating and running to the bathroom immediately after eating had ruined her social life—preventing her from dating or even going on casual lunches with friends. She confessed that her friends would sometimes call her when

---

1. Healthlink, "Celiac Disease," Medical College of Wisconsin, http://healthlink.mcw.edu/article/956622658.html.

they were traveling, as they knew she had an intimate knowledge of the best and worst bathrooms along the I–40 corridor. She described how her condition had worsened to the point that her doctor finally removed her gall bladder, leaving her feeling worse than ever. She had no health insurance and this surgery had severely depleted her financial resources, not to mention her mental and physical health.

No one in the course of all of her various medical visits had ever mentioned the words *celiac disease* to her and yet here she and her father stood, informed by a simple phone call from a friend the day before about a disease that very likely affected many members of their family. My heart ached for her and for all she had lost in the time she had been suffering, but I was also filled with hope for her and for her family, that they would soon have answers that would give them their lives back. Knowing how much better life can be for a celiac when correctly diagnosed and living comfortably on a gluten-free diet, it is truly hard for me to contain my enthusiasm for educating others like them on the chance that my information might change their lives for the better.

I never diagnose anyone with CD and take great pains to explain to people that I am in no way qualified to make such diagnoses, but I strongly urge those whom I suspect of having it to see their physician right away for testing.

In your daily life, contemplate whether sharing information about your diagnosis might filter down to another who was previously unaware of the disease. Even if it does not eventually help to educate a person who has undiagnosed celiac disease, consider that it might help a waiter or a restaurateur more carefully handle the next meal ordered by a patron with CD or other food intolerance. Speaking directly with those in the food service industry about your dietary needs—adding in the details of how many other potential patrons have similar restrictions—can go a long way toward causing those restaurants to begin to offer additional safe alternatives for celiacs. Restaurateurs are business people like any others, who are interested in hearing from their customer base. Become friendly with the staff at a select number of restaurants and frequent them, educating them by sharing your restrictions and offering your suggestions. You will be surprised at how willing many of these restaurants will be to accommodate your needs and to modify their menus to attract others like you, once they understand that there is an established demand for gluten-free food.

Keeping your health information private is of course your prerogative. However, I believe that we all have an obligation to spread the word about CD until the medical community and the population at large are familiar enough with it to properly diagnose it. Making our voices heard helps others learn of the disease to be sure, but it also gives others a more accurate picture of how many of us there are in the world. We are a market that needs to be served, a demand that needs to be answered, and a large group that deserves to be understood and not isolated. The more our voices are heard, the more all will learn about themselves and about us.

◇ ◇ ◇

Spread the Word: S. Drew's Story

I discovered that I had celiac disease when I read the book *Eat Right for Your Type*, which cautioned that a person with blood type O should not eat wheat. I stopped eating wheat and was suddenly healthy. Before that time, I was very sick all the time. Twenty-three years earlier, the doctor just told me my problem was an idiosyncrasy of my body. I was sick every day and was unable to discern what caused my problem. Eventually the doctor even took out my gallbladder; some of my sickness was alleviated, but I was still sick most days.

Now I have to tell you I am very positive about my diagnosis with celiac disease. I celebrate that I am not sick any longer. I can now travel, hike, exercise, and really do most anything I would choose. I see myself as a much healthier eater. I eat mesquite flour, tapioca flour, soy flour, brown rice flour, just to name a few, which I see as much healthier than the man-made wheat flour. Furthermore, I like to be able to tell someone, "I can not eat that." So many times people want you to eat something that is not good for you and I actually have a good excuse to avoid sugared or fatty treats. I figure I am eating many fewer fat calories and sugar-sweetened calories, so I celebrate my disease for that reason as well.

When I go to a restaurant and ask all my questions, I figure I am educating another person about celiac. Besides, when people ask questions, I am glad to tell them about my symptoms. Just maybe they have the same disease and have been sick for many years, too. Or just as important, maybe they know someone else that may have celiac and a doctor who also thinks it is an idiosyncrasy of their body.

One of my current jobs is as a coordinator for Elderhostel. Participants often notice that my meals can be quite different than theirs. Often I find myself explaining why I do not eat bread. Again, maybe they are having the same problems or know someone else with the same symptoms. Many times a participant has said, "I wonder if that is what my friend has—she has been very sick for years with similar symptoms."

Some of my in-laws have had health problems as well. I kept educating them about my symptoms and suggest that they, too, try a gluten-free diet. Now three family members have joined me and they are symptom free and feel so much healthier. I feel good knowing I have helped them feel better, too.

I realize that if you are not feeding your body properly, your body will not have the nutrition to function properly. Since doctors do not seem to test for celiac or even know about celiac, patients have to realize their own problems and present that problem to the doctor. This makes it even more important to talk about celiac disease with others.

◇ ◇ ◇

IN A SENTENCE

Sharing (not preaching) information about celiac disease can help others find treatment, but the best way to help others is to carefully preserve the delicate balance between educating and diagnosing.

living

A Blessing in Disguise:
Kathleen Barrett's Story

WHILE WE can all benefit from the many rapid medical advances being made in the realm of celiac disease, some have taken the need for more research and more skilled clinicians to heart on an even more personal level. Kathleen Barrett changed career paths entirely after her diagnosis with CD and dedicated her life to helping others through medicine.

◇ ◇ ◇

Kathleen Barrett's Story

By the time I was diagnosed with celiac disease in 1997, I would have eaten bananas and Jell-O the rest of my life if that was what it took to get rid of the pain, diarrhea, and bloating. I immediately threw out all the bread, soups, and bagels and started over, which included more than just my diet. I created a new outlook.

I started researching celiac disease on my own. I soon discovered it was not well-known, very little research was being done, and there was no magic cure. In fact, after trying to return to work too soon after diagnosis, my body was too weak and I was forced to go on medical disability. Even the insurance company denied my claim for one year, stating "celiac spruce" (yes, they called it *spruce* like the tree, not *sprue* as in diarrhea) was not a legitimate reason to be ill enough to miss work, despite the fact that I had heard stories of people starving in nursing homes and hospitals because no one knew how to feed them.

The turning point came when a few short months later, a newly diagnosed celiac was on the phone asking *me* for help. That was when it changed my life's focus. Instead of going back to my public relations job, when I was finally able to work again, I decided to go to medical school. The two things needed most were research and raising awareness, both in the general and medical communities.

It was a long hard road, but in August 2003 I enrolled at the University of Maryland School of Medicine. At the beginning of my second year, my body starting shutting down as it had when I was first diagnosed with celiac. This time, it was autoimmune thyroid issues that had originally surfaced six months after the celiac diagnosis. I had to take leave from school and move home to Chicago for a few months so my parents could take care of me. I was thirty-one years old, experiencing the second yearlong medical leave of my life and the second need to move back with my parents because my body could barely function. My world had fallen down around me and I was crushed to step out of the common path that almost all other med students take: to finish in four years.

But eight months later, as I rejoined my new class at the start of second year, I discovered it was yet another blessing in disguise. I was healthier than ever, more focused, and my new classmates were welcoming and accepting. I soon found a new group of lifelong friends to add to the ones from my previous class. Sure, it is hard when all the free lunches in the school and hospital are pizza, sandwiches, or pasta, but I am always prepared with my lunch and get a pleasant surprise if what is being provided is something I can actually eat. And honestly, I have had fewer celiac episodes in med school without the time or money to eat out as much.

I spent several months on the road interviewing for residency positions around the Midwest and up and down the East Coast. I stocked up on my favorite gluten-free power bars, trail mix, and fruit, and even some Danishes from the gluten-free bakery here in Baltimore, to fit right in with the other applicants at the continental breakfasts. Lunch was often an adventure but only once did I become sick from the hidden croutons in the salad.

Through all of this, I've become a planner. Yet all I need is a few food items in a bag, and I can still be as spontaneous as I used to be. My other discovery is probably the greatest. People are kind and accommodating and willing to make exceptions if they know the reason. As long as you are doing your best with what you have and making the most out of every situation, they will do the same for you.

As I look back now, just a few months shy of my graduation from medical school, I remember that I never would have decided to become a doctor if it weren't for being diagnosed with celiac disease. And I also realize how much has changed. Almost anyone I ask has heard of celiac disease or knows someone who has it, the food options are more plentiful and much more appealing, and several clinical and research centers around the country have discovered more about this disease than ever thought possible. They are even developing drugs now to allow us to eat a certain amount of gluten. Every celiac has made this journey and is more than willing to help someone who is newly diagnosed. Ask for help, educate those around you, and look for the things you *can* do and the things you *can* eat in every situation.

◇ ◇ ◇

IN A SENTENCE

You can view your celiac diagnosis as a limiting event, or as an opportunity to open new doors.

MONTH 5

Celiac and Infertility

MANY WOMEN first learn of their celiac disease in the course of their attempts to become pregnant. Up to 7.4 percent of all married women aged fifteen to forty-four years of age are **infertile** (that is, they are not surgically sterile, have not used contraception in the past twelve months, but have not become pregnant). Even more stunning is the statistic that over 25 percent of married childless women aged fifteen to forty-four have **impaired fecundity** (in other words, they are not surgically sterile yet it is nonetheless difficult or impossible to get pregnant or to carry a pregnancy to term.)[1] A significant proportion of unfavorable pregnancy outcomes have no specific cause, yet celiac disease is now considered to be one of the systemic disorders that could account for a large percentage of unexplained infertility and impaired fecundity. Many studies have shown that as many as 6 percent of infertile women are undiagnosed celiacs.[2] CD is

---

1. National Center for Health Statistics, "Key Statistics from the NSFG," Centers for Disease Control and Prevention (2002), http://www.cdc.gov/nchs/about/major/nsfg/abclist_i.htm#infertility.
2. Stephano Guandalini, MD, "Celiac Disease Does Not Cause Infertility in the U.S. or Does It?" *Impact* 8, no. 1 (Winter 2008): 1–2.

now well recognized as the root cause of many women's infertility, but also of male infertility, delayed menarche (initiation of the menstrual cycle), amenorrhea (cessation of the menstrual cycle for various periods of time), early menopause, and even sexual dysfunction.[3]

Recent international research has demonstrated what many have argued for all along: that celiac disease should be routinely screened for in all cases of unexplained infertility or unfavorable pregnancy outcomes such as spontaneous abortion, miscarriage, low-birth-weight babies, preterm deliveries, and stillbirths. Undiagnosed CD is more common than most all the widely screened conditions that may lead to these unfavorable events. A major study in Italy concluded that as many as 1 in 70 women was affected by celiac disease (CD is more prevalent in women than in men), which led directly to a range of negative pregnancy outcomes. Because CD is easily treatable through diet, the study was also able to demonstrate treating these women with a gluten-free diet remarkably improved fertility and reduced or eliminated unfavorable outcomes of pregnancy.[4]

If you and your doctor believe that celiac disease might be the root cause of your infertility or fecundity problems, you should waste no time in being

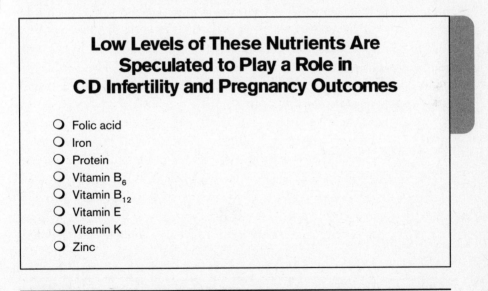

Low Levels of These Nutrients Are Speculated to Play a Role in CD Infertility and Pregnancy Outcomes

○ Folic acid
○ Iron
○ Protein
○ Vitamin B_6
○ Vitamin B_{12}
○ Vitamin E
○ Vitamin K
○ Zinc

3. K. Rostami et al., "Coeliac Disease and Reproductive Disorders: A Neglected Association," *European Journal of Obstetrics & Gynocology and Reproductive Biology* 96, no. 2 (June 2001): 146–49.

4. P. Martinelli et al., "Cœliac Disease and Unfavorable Outcome of Pregnancy," *Gut* 46 (2000): 332–35.

tested—both serologically and endoscopically—for CD. Remember that trying a gluten-free diet in advance of any testing will impair the accuracy of these tests, so do not undertake a gluten-free diet prior to any such tests. If a diagnosis of celiac disease is ultimately made, then an appointment with a nutritionist specializing in gluten-free diets or with a gluten-free expert should be your top priority. Consulting with an expert in gluten-free living—cooking, shopping, and eating out—will put you on the path to good health and hopefully to a healthy pregnancy that much sooner.

If You Are Pregnant

If you are already pregnant and celiac disease is suspected from a history of miscarriages, anemia, low-birth-weight babies, other unfavorable outcomes with pregnancies, or other symptoms, celiac serology should be ordered. If those tests are positive, however, a biopsy would need to be postponed until after the baby is born and nursing has ceased. In the meantime, you should immediately adopt a strict gluten-free diet until such time as your physician determines you can undergo a gluten challenge followed by an endoscopic biopsy. It could be extremely detrimental to both you and your fetus if, as a celiac, you fail to adhere to a strict gluten-free diet during pregnancy; a healthy gluten-free diet will provide all the nutritional requirements your fetus will need in the womb.[5] You may choose not to do a gluten-challenge, and in that case, you should undertake genetic testing to confirm compatibility with celiac disease.[6]

IN A SENTENCE

Celiac disease should be considered as a possible cause for unexplained infertility, even if there are no other overt symptoms; if you learn that you have celiac disease, a gluten-free diet should return your body and your fertility to a normal range.

5. Michelle Melin-Rogovin, "Fertility and Pregnancy in Women with Celiac Disease," Celiac.com, http://www.celiac.com/articles/643/1/Fertility-and-Pregnancy-in-Women-with-Celiac-Disease-by-Michelle-Melin-Rogovin/Page1.html.
6. Stephano Guandalini, MD, "Celiac Disease Does Not Cause Infertility in the U.S. or Does It?" *Impact* 8, no. 1 (Winter 2008): 1–2.

living

Discovering You're Celiac after Pregnancy

ONCE YOU achieve a successful pregnancy, it is imperative that you continue to listen to your body and remain strictly gluten-free. Adopting a gluten-free diet will help both you and your baby cope with the challenges that are inevitable with any new little family member in your life.

Often, though, the physical stress of a pregnancy actually tips the balance for women genetically predisposed to celiac disease, and active CD begins during or shortly after pregnancy. If your health during this time leads you to suspect celiac disease might be causing your symptoms, you should seek immediate serological and potentially endoscopic testing. You cannot afford— particularly during this emotionally and physically stressful time after the birth of your baby—to have your health in jeopardy.

Tanya Hanshew, like many celiac women, only discovered that she had CD after a seemingly healthy pregnancy deteriorated her body and ushered in a host of physical ailments. Fortunately, after diagnosis and beginning a gluten-free diet, she and her children are now happy and healthy.

◇ ◇ ◇

New Baby + New Diagnosis = Healthy Future:
Tanya Hanshew's Story

When I was a child with undiagnosed celiac disease, I experienced many health issues, the most poignant memories being painful muscle cramps in my legs and stomach, and being forced to drink Metamucil to cure constipation. Because our family moved many times in my young years, pediatricians were not able to piece together the symptoms for a correct diagnosis. During my teen years, I was very petite and didn't get my period until age fifteen. Throughout my early adulthood, diagnoses included fibromyalgia, rheumatoid arthritis, anemia, and irritable bowel syndrome, for which they prescribed a high-fiber diet consisting of whole grains. Anathema to a celiac!

At age twenty-seven, I found out that my husband and I were expecting our first child. With great anticipation and excitement, we looked forward to welcoming the new baby to our lives. My pregnancy symptoms were minimal and, other than some annoying heartburn in the last trimester, the nine months were quite uncomplicated. Morgan was born in mid-January at a healthy 8 pounds 13 ounces, but shortly after arriving home I noticed changes occurring in my health.

I began breast-feeding in the hospital, but after one week Morgan had not gained an ounce and the doctors began to encourage me to supplement her feedings. As a dedicated new mom, I was willing to do whatever was necessary to give my baby the best start, namely, breast-feeding. And so I made an appointment with the lactation consultant and completed the evaluation process. To her credit, the consultant was informative, encouraging, and thorough and concluded that it had to be a milk-supply issue. To increase my milk supply, I rented a hospital-grade breast pump, began pumping, took doses of fenugreek, supplemented Morgan with a feeding tube system of extra, pumped milk after breast-feeding, and set my alarm clock at two-hour intervals for nighttime feedings. Between nursing, pumping, and supplemental feedings, I was spending twelve hours a day just feeding my newborn daughter. I felt incredible guilt and sadness about not being able to breast-feed successfully and tried so hard to figure out what the problem was. Little did I know that it had to do with my health—there was nothing I was doing wrong.

While I was somewhat consumed with helping Morgan grow, my physical health was overlooked. The reality was that I was rapidly losing weight, having uncontrollable diarrhea, and experiencing depression. The first few weeks after having your first baby should ideally be warm, sweet, and memorable—a time for bonding between baby and mom. But mine was not. Unbeknownst to me, my celiac disease was now in a fully active stage. My abdominal pain was constant and, some days, it was even difficult to leave the house because of cramping. It can only be described as pure torment.

After eight weeks of struggling to breast-feed, I began bottle-feeding Morgan. Almost instantly, her demeanor changed from one of discontentment to complete satisfaction. I still remember the first full bottle I gave her of formula, crying the whole time I fed her, thinking I was a failure. Then, miraculously, she began sleeping through the night.

In the meantime, my negligent physician prescribed antidepressants and told me I was just an anxious new mom. He even told me on one particular visit that I was nothing short of a hypochondriac. Around this time, two of my sisters were visiting for a few days. My older sister returned home after seeing how sick I was, began researching my varied symptoms, and convinced me to see a gastroenterologist. Finally, within one month, I was diagnosed with celiac disease. I quickly made changes to my diet, and within days the pain was subsiding and energy was increasing. After just two months on a gluten-free diet, my iron levels were healthy and I was beginning to gain weight (my prepregnancy weight had been about 128; at the height of my illness, it was down to 112).

Twelve months after our daughter was born and just three months after being diagnosed, I became pregnant again. We were excited and since my health was steadily improving, there was no reason to be concerned. Our second daughter was born at a healthy eight and a half pounds. I attempted to breast-feed her for several weeks but when she wasn't gaining steadily, decided to switch to formula. This time, there was no guilt as I gave up breast-feeding and realized that both my daughters were healthy and had received the best of what I could give them—my love. They are very healthy children and have had steady growth; neither of them experienced a single ear infection in their first year and, other than catching a winter cold, have not been seriously ill. I have had my oldest daughter tested for CD (negative) and will soon have my youngest daughter tested, although neither shows any physical signs of illness to date.

◇ ◇ ◇

IN A SENTENCE

Pregnancy already brings about many physical and psychological changes for moms, add newly active celiac disease to the mix and things get even more complicated; if you ignore your bodily changes during this stressful time, you may risk not only your health, but that of your new baby.

Entertaining and Being Entertained

So now that you've mastered making your own food in your own home, as well as venturing out to restaurants for special meals, how do you attend social events at another person's home safely without either martyring yourself by not eating anything at all, or embarrassing others who kindly but unsuccessfully try to prepare gluten-free food for you?

When You're the Guest

Obviously, the generic party invitation is not too much of an issue. You simply eat beforehand and nibble on the vegetable tray (without dipping into the ranch dressing) as you mingle and socialize. It is always polite to bring a bottle of wine with you as a guest, and at least that would be something you might be able to enjoy with the host as well. A dinner party may pose a number of other problems—but solvable ones.

Clearly, your good friends and family will have you over no matter what the circumstances, they may be well versed in the art of gluten-free cooking, and they would probably love for you to bring a yummy gluten-free dish. However, things can become trickier when you are not close friends with your host or hostess. Unless I know the hosts very well, I often do not want to disclose my dietary restrictions so that they don't feel they must go out of their way to try to make something special for me to eat. More often than not, if they do make something gluten-free, it is either unappetizing or really not entirely gluten-free. As you know by now, learning to live gluten-free takes some time and effort. How can one honestly expect someone who is not used to cooking this way and not a paid cooking professional to similarly master the sometimes obscure lists of hidden glutens while preparing to host a non-gluten-free party? What I have instead learned is the subtle art of gluten-free etiquette (a.k.a. "How to remain on the guest list at non-gluten-free parties"!).

From here, it is all about what you are comfortable with saying and how much. Your response to the wife of your husband's largest client will probably be somewhat different from what you say to your book club's newest member. The most effective approach I have learned is to graciously accept the offer while simultaneously asking what you can bring as a contribution. You can take it from there and explain as much or as little as you want about celiac disease or dietary restrictions. Since the most difficult conversation is the one wherein your object is to disclose as little as possible about yourself, that is the approach taken in the hypothetical conversations outlined below.

Handling a Party Invitation 101:

YOU: We would be happy to join you! What can I bring to the party?

HOST: "Thank you for offering; that would be wonderful. Just bring whatever you want."

YOU: "Great! What are you serving, so I can be sure to bring something that will complement the rest of your meal? [*thinking: Yay! I'm home free because I can bring a main dish, bread, casserole—whatever I want to eat, and now she is going to tell me in advance what other food options I might have!*]

or

HOST: "Thank you for offering, why don't you bring an appetizer?"

YOU: "I'd be happy to. What else are you serving, so I can be sure to bring something that will complement the rest of your meal as well?" [*thinking: Fine, I'll bring an appetizer, find out from her in advance what else I might be able to eat, and I'll still show up with gluten-free bread or a casse-role or whatever else I want to have to eat in addition!"*]

or

HOST: "No, thanks. I've got it covered!"

YOU: "Wow, you are ambitious—I can't wait to enjoy a night out with some-one else cooking! What are you planning on serving? . . . How about I bring a [*fill in the blank with something you like*] to complement that dish? I've really been wanting to try this delicious new recipe, and it will give me a chance to make it and get your opinion on it."

or

HOST: "No, it's being catered, so there's nothing to worry about!"

YOU: "Fantastic! I can't wait! Who are you having do the catering?/What will they be serving?" [*Then you call the caterer and ask details about the ingredients.*]

If instead, you feel comfortable informing your host or hostess about celiac disease and gluten-free foods, the conversation will flow even more easily. (See Month 4 for the ways and reasons for discussing celiac disease with others.) You can use this as an opportunity to not only expand his or her culinary horizons but also to expose this individual to information on celiac disease that might ultimately help someone else who has not yet been diagnosed. Be careful not to preach, though, and keep the conversation as light as you can, emphasizing all the positives and the many yummy things those on a gluten-free diet may still enjoy. Whatever you do, never forget to thank the host or hostess for his or her interest and concern for your dietary needs. There often is no substitute for a handwritten thank-you note.

Hosting Parties

One approach to prevent a dance around the ingredient list is to host parties yourself, whenever possible. You are then in control of the meal and the preparation area, you know that you are safe, and now you know how to pre-pare delicious foods that others will enjoy as well. Potlucks are wonderful party ideas, in this case. Many people who are unfamiliar with the gluten-free diet (or are familiar with the old-school way of cooking gluten-free) will be hesitant to come for dinner if they know that you are cooking gluten-free and think they won't enjoy gluten-free food. I liken this trepidation to the days when I was just a vegetarian (now I'm a seafood-eating vegetarian celiac—much more complicated!) and some carnivorous friends interpreted my dinner-party invites as an invitation to eat tofu and sprouts. Sadly mistaken as they were, they learned after actually attending my dinners that the realm of good vegetarian food is far more broad and delicious. Easing these kinds of folks into the idea of a gluten-free meal is made much more palatable by suggesting that everyone bring a dish to contribute and to share with the other guests even if you can't taste the dish yourself. Once they are at the dinner and taste your dishes, they will know that next time, they will gladly eat your gluten-free food without reservation.

The next section is dedicated to providing you with perfect recipes to serve at dinner parties (or bring to a friend's). These recipes are tried and true favorites of celiacs and nonceliacs alike; you can proudly and safely serve them yourself. Just make sure to bring enough for everyone!

IN A SENTENCE

> *There are many easy ways to deftly respond to social invitations while still participating and enjoying yourself; gluten-free limitations do not have to restrict your social life any more than you let them.*

living

Gluten-Free
Recipes for a Crowd

AS JUST discussed, one way to handle social situations involving food is to prepare your own, either to bring to a party or to serve as the host. Enjoy some of these fabulous recipes at your next social occasion and don't even bother telling folks these dishes are gluten-free—the guests will never know!

Appetizers and Munchies

Hot Spinach and Artichoke Dip

THIS IS a great, already typically gluten-free party favorite served with corn tortilla chips. The recipe can easily be doubled by using two pie pans or one 9 by 13-inch casserole.

Serves 10

1 (14-ounce) can artichoke hearts, drained and mashed

10 ounces frozen, thawed, and drained or fresh spinach, chopped

1 cup Miracle Whip salad dressing or mayonnaise

1 cup grated Parmesan cheese

Minced garlic or garlic powder (to taste)

Minced green onions or tomatoes (optional)

1. Preheat the oven to 350°F.
2. Mix all the ingredients together, adding minced garlic or garlic powder to taste, and spoon into a 9-inch pie plate. Bake for 45 minutes, until lightly browned on top. Sprinkle with chopped green onions or tomatoes, if desired, and serve warm.

Mango Salsa

THIS FRESH salsa is amazing, served with corn tortilla chips or as a topping for grilled fish or chicken. Guests ask for this recipe every time I bring it to summer parties; it is refreshing, light, and unusual enough to make an impression.

Serves 6

1 fresh, ripe mango, pitted and diced

$1/2$ cup seeded and diced red bell pepper

$1/4$ cup diced red onion

$1/2$ teaspoon ground cumin

$1/4$ teaspoon Tabasco sauce

1 tablespoon fresh lime juice or True Lime

1 teaspoon chopped fresh cilantro (optional)

Mix all ingredients in a bowl and refrigerate until serving.

Maryland Crab Balls

THE OLD Bay Seasoning is a must to make these mini crab cakes worthy of the Maryland moniker. You won't even miss the bread crumbs—I promise! The key to successful crab dishes of any kind is always to buy quality lump crabmeat. Do not skimp on this step, or no crab dish, no matter how many bread crumbs, is worthy of serving to guests.

Serves 8

1 pound high-quality lump crabmeat, cleaned and drained

1 1/3 cups crushed corn tortilla chips, plus extra crushed chips, for dredging

1/3 cup minced green onions

1/3 cup chopped fresh parsley

2 tablespoons lemon juice

1 tablespoon milk

1 teaspoon Tabasco or other hot sauce

1/2 teaspoon salt

1/4 teaspoon pepper

4 eggs

Old Bay Seasoning

Olive oil

Gluten-free crackers (I recommend Hol-Grain brand or other gluten-free rice crackers)

Romaine lettuce leaves

1. In a bowl, combine the crabmeat, the 1 1/3 cups crushed tortilla chips, green onions, parsley, lemon juice, milk, hot sauce, salt, pepper, eggs, and Old Bay Seasoning. Mix well with a fork. Divide this mixture into sixteen equal portions, roll into small balls or patties, and dredge thoroughly with the additional crushed tortilla chips.

2. To grill, wrap each crabmeat ball individually in foil and cook for approximately 5 minutes on each side. To broil, place on oiled baking sheet and broil for approximately 5 minutes per side. To fry, heat enough olive oil to cover at least 1/8 inch deep in a large skillet at medium-high heat. Place the patties in the hot oil and cook for 3 minutes on each side, or roll the balls around in the oil to cook on all sides.

3. Serve on gluten-free crackers with a small piece of lettuce under each ball.

Salty and Sweet Party Mix

ASIDE FROM setting out gluten-free pretzels (many of which, such as Glutino brand, are pretty darn good) or a bowl of nuts, sometimes it's just nice to have a snack mix to offer, particularly at a nondinner party where there is a lot of milling about or children present. I have found that this mix is enjoyed by everyone, as it so closely matches the famous "Chex Mix" we all find synonymous with football games and parties. Another option is simply to follow these directions to candy the pecans and set them out as a dish unto themselves. Yum!

Makes 9 cups

1/4 cup butter or nondairy alternative

2 cups halved pecans

1/8 cup granulated cane sugar

1 1/2 cups gluten-free pretzel sticks (such as Glutino brand)

1 1/2 cups pretzel twists (such as Glutino brand)

2 cups General Mills Rice Chex cereal[1] or Health Valley Rice (or Corn) Crunch-Ems

1 cup salted cashews or mixed nuts

1 cup white or dark chocolate chips

1. Melt the butter in a skillet over low heat and lightly brown the pecans. Add the sugar, stirring until the sugar is dissolved and the pecans are slightly shiny. Pour the pecans onto a cookie sheet lined with paper towels. Spread the pecans over the paper towels, pat, then pour onto another unlined cookie sheet to cool (do not let cool on the paper towels or the nuts will stick to the towels).

2. Place the cooled nuts and all the other ingredients in a large bowl, mix, and serve. Store in sealed zip-top bags.

---

1. In the spring of 2008, General Mills announced that it had reformulated its Rice Chex cereal to no longer include barley malt extract. Instead, sugar and molasses are the added sweeteners to this now gluten-free cereal. So far, Corn Chex is still not gluten-free, as barley malt extract remains on its ingredient label. For more information see http://www.bellinstitute.com/wic/topic/section_detail.aspx?cat_1 =200&selectCatID=200&catID=200&itemID=6173.

Spinach Dip with a Kick

THIS RECIPE has that Southern spicy flair that makes it an out-of-the-ordinary dip. The secret is in the chiles and the Tabasco sauce. It is a real crowd-pleaser when served with corn tortilla chips.

Serves 6

2 (10-ounce) packages frozen spinach

8 ounces cream cheese (light works fine, too)

2 cups shredded Monterey Jack cheese

2 (10-ounce) can Rotel, or 1 (4.5-ounce) can chopped green chiles plus 1 (14.5-ounce) can or 2 cups fresh chopped tomatoes

1 cup half-and-half or whipping cream

Tabasco sauce

1. Preheat the oven to 350°F. Grease a 9 by 13-inch oblong baking dish.

2. Rinse the spinach until it is thawed and broken apart. Place it with all the remaining ingredients, except the Tabasco, in a large bowl and mix well with an electric mixer. Add splashes of Tabasco sauce until it suits your taste. Pour into the prepared baking dish and bake for 10 minutes, or until the cheese has melted and the top is lightly browned.

3. Serve with corn or tortilla chips.

Side Dishes

Rice con Queso

THIS RECIPE may also serve as a main dish, particularly if there are vegetarians in your midst. Brown or white rice works equally well here.

Serves 6

1 cup cooked rice

1 (15-ounce) can black beans, drained and rinsed

$1/2$ cup chopped green chiles, (1 small can)

$1/4$ cup chopped onion

$1/4$ teaspoon ground cumin

$1/4$ teaspoon ground coriander

$1/2$ teaspoon salt

1 cup light or whole-milk ricotta cheese

$1/3$ cup milk

2 cups shredded Monterey Jack or Cheddar Jack cheese

1. Preheat the oven to 350°F. Grease an 8-inch square baking pan.

2. Pour the cooked rice into a large mixing bowl. Add the black beans, chopped chilies, onions, and spices, and mix together well.

3. In a small bowl, mix together the ricotta cheese, milk, and $1 1/2$ cups of the shredded cheese. Add the cheese mixture to the rice and stir.

4. Pour the entire mixture into the prepared baking pan and bake for 20 minutes. Sprinkle the remaining shredded cheese on top and bake for an additional 10 minutes.

Sweet Potato Casserole

THIS IS a fantastic recipe to take to a potluck dinner. The texture from the grated sweet potatoes makes this dish unique.

Serves 8

1 cup sugar

3 eggs, beaten

1 (12-ounce) can evaporated milk

1 teaspoon gluten-free vanilla extract

$\frac{1}{4}$ cup melted butter

1 cup milk

$\frac{1}{2}$ teaspoon ground ginger

1 teaspoon ground cinnamon

$1\frac{1}{2}$ cups peeled and grated sweet potatoes

1. Beat all the ingredients except the sweet potatoes in a large bowl. Stir in the sweet potatoes. Pour mixture into an ungreased 9 by 13-inch pan and place in a cold oven. Bake at 325°F for 1 hour.

Main Dishes

Crab and Asparagus Mini Casseroles

THIS IS a fun recipe to serve at a dinner gathering, as each couple can share a mini casserole as part of the meal! I have offered some suggested alternative ingredients, but this recipe is one in which other substituted veggies would work well, too.

**Serves 4 to 8, depending on what other
dishes are offered for the main course.**

1 bunch fresh, steamed asparagus

1/4 cup finely chopped onion

1 tablespoon butter or nondairy substitute

1 cup sliced fresh mushrooms

1 tablespoon finely ground nuts such as almonds or pecans, or cornstarch

Pinch of salt

Pinch of black pepper

Pinch of grated nutmeg

1 cup milk (skim or nondairy is fine)

1/2 cup shredded mozzarella cheese or nondairy alternative

8 ounces high-quality lump crabmeat, cleaned and drained

2 tablespoons chopped toasted almonds

2 tablespoons fresh grated Parmesan or Asiago cheese (do not use if preparing this recipe dairy-free)

Extra-virgin olive oil

1. Preheat the oven to 400°F. Oil four small ramekins. This is important, as the mixture becomes too watery if it is all combined into one large casserole.

2. Steam and drain the asparagus; cut the spears into bite-size chunks and set aside.

3. In a medium-size skillet, sauté the onions in the butter until the onions are tender but not yet browned.

4. Add and cook the mushrooms.

5. Next, add the ground nuts, salt, pepper, and nutmeg. After mixing well, stir in the milk over medium-low heat, until thickened and bubbly. Cook, stirring, for 1 minute more, then add the mozzarella cheese, crabmeat, and asparagus.

6. Divide the mixture among the four ramekins. Sprinkle the tops with an equal amount of toasted almonds and cheese.

8. Bake for 10 minutes, or until the cheese topping is browned. Serve warm.

Creole Crabmeat Casserole

I AM always searching for meals I can prepare and serve for days to come. This casserole is like many that gets better after sitting for even one day—a bonus if you are throwing a party and need to make some food ahead of time! Feel free to add more seasoning, but the recipe provides a nice flavor as it is. I am always amazed at how easy this recipe is, yet how deliciously difficult it looks when prepared. After I shared this simple recipe in my first cookbook, several blogs have praised its virtues.

Serves 8

8 ounces high-quality lump crabmeat, cleaned and drained

1$\frac{1}{2}$ cups instant, uncooked rice

1 onion, chopped

$\frac{1}{2}$ green, orange, yellow, or red bell pepper, seeded, or to taste

1 (10$\frac{1}{2}$-ounce) can gluten-free tomato soup

2 tablespoons olive oil

2 tablespoons Worcestershire sauce

1 teaspoon Tabasco sauce, or to taste

1 teaspoon salt

8 ounces fresh or canned chopped and seeded tomatoes

Shredded cheese (optional)

1. Preheat the oven to 325°F. Oil a casserole dish.

2. Combine all the ingredients in a bowl and place in the prepared casserole dish. Cover with foil and bake for 35 minutes. You may add shredded cheese and cook, uncovered for an additional 5 minutes, if you prefer.

Mexican Lasagne

THIS NOODLE-FREE recipe is a fun twist on an old traditional dish. If you do not care for gluten-free rice lasagna noodles, this is a great way to have your lasagne and celiac, too!

Serves 8

1 pound lean ground beef, ground turkey, or firm tofu

1/2 cup chopped onion

1/2 cup seeded and chopped green, orange, or sweet red bell pepper

2 1/2 cups chunky salsa

1 (8 3/4-ounce) can corn, drained, or 2 ears cooked corn, cut off cob

1 teaspoon chile powder

1 teaspoon ground cumin

10 corn tortillas, cut in half

2 cups (16 ounces) small-curd cottage cheese (Lactaid brand has a lactose-free version) or ricotta cheese

1 cup shredded sharp Cheddar cheese or nondairy alternative

2 small cans sliced, pitted ripe olives, drained (optional)

1. Preheat the oven to 350°F.

2. Brown the meat, onion, and pepper in a large skillet over medium heat, then drain. Add the salsa, corn, and seasonings. Layer one-third of the meat sauce, half the tortillas, and half the cottage cheese in a 9 by 13-inch baking dish. Repeat the layers, ending with meat sauce. Sprinkle with Cheddar cheese and olives, if using. Bake for 30 minutes.

Desserts

Family Fudge

MY MOTHER has been making this recipe since I was a little girl, and she has modified it to fit modern kitchens by creating a microwave version (which is much easier!). Variations you may want to try include using peanut butter chips instead of chocolate chips, putting crushed candy canes or colored sugar on top, or adding nuts to the fudge. No candy thermometer needed!

Serves 10

3 cups sugar

12 tablespoons (1$^1\!/_2$ sticks) butter or margarine

5 ounces evaporated milk (fat-free is fine)

1 jar marshmallow cream

12 ounces semisweet chocolate chips

1 teaspoon vanilla extract

1 cup chopped nuts (optional)

1. Place the sugar, butter, and evaporated milk in a large, microwave-safe bowl and microwave on high until melted. Stir, then microwave until the mixture comes to a full rolling boil. Without turning the microwave off or opening the door, add 5 minutes of boiling time to microwaving the mixture.

2. Meanwhile, oil a 9 by 13-inch baking pan. Open the jar of marshmallow cream and the bag of chocolate chips, so that they are ready to add immediately after the boiling process is completed.

3. Scoop the marshmallow cream and pour the chips into the boiling mixture and stir vigorously to mix. Add the vanilla extract and nuts, if using, then use a mixer to beat the mixture until smooth. Quickly pour into the prepared pan and smooth, using a rubber or silicone spatula. Add any toppings you desire at this point, then set aside to cool. Do not cut until the fudge has cooled (usually at least 1 to 2 hours).

Lemon Bars

LEMON IS a flavor I can never get enough of after a meal. It is the perfect conclusion to practically any dinner, so it goes well at parties. This bar can be cut and eaten as a finger food.

Makes 20 bars.
This recipe doubles nicely when baked in a 9 by 13-inch pan.

Crust

$\frac{1}{3}$ cup butter or nondairy alternative

$\frac{1}{4}$ cup granulated sugar

1 cup Nearly Normal All-Purpose Flour (page 48)

Filling

2 eggs

$\frac{3}{4}$ cup granulated sugar

2 tablespoons Nearly Normal All-Purpose Flour (page 48)

2 teaspoons finely shredded lemon zest

3 tablespoons lemon juice, or $\frac{3}{4}$ teaspoon True Lemon powder
reconstituted in 3 tablespoons water

$\frac{1}{4}$ teaspoon gluten-free baking powder

Confectioners' sugar, for dusting (optional)

1. Preheat the oven to 350°F.

2. Prepare the crust: In a medium-size bowl, beat the butter with an electric mixer at medium to high speed for 30 seconds. Add the sugar; beat until combined. Beat in the flour mixture until crumbly, being careful not to over-mix. Press the dough into the bottom of an ungreased 8-inch square baking pan. Bake for 15 minutes, or until golden.

3. Prepare the filling: Combine the eggs, sugar, flour mixture, lemon zest, lemon juice, and baking powder in a medium-size bowl; beat for 2 minutes or until combined.

4. Pour the filling over the baked crust. Bake for 20 more minutes, or until set and lightly browned. Cool on a wire rack. Cut into bars when completely cool. (Sprinkle with confectioners' sugar before serving, if desired.)

Peanut Butter Crispy Rice Treats

WE ALL grew up loving "Rice Krispies Treats" but now have been denied even such a simple pleasure unless we make them ourselves using gluten-free cereal (Warning: This means you cannot use Kellogg's Rice Krispies because it contains malt flavoring!). Fortunately, such an option is available and just as delicious. I add peanut butter chips to my recipe for added flavor; straight peanut butter tends to make the treats mushy after they cool. My kids also like to add seasonally colored sugar and gluten-free sprinkles to make the treats more festive.

Serves 15

3 tablespoons butter or nondairy alternative

4 cups miniature marshmallows

6 cups gluten-free crispy rice cereal (Do *not* use puffy rice cereal. Nature's Path and Erewhon make two good crispy rice cereal options)

$1/2$ cup peanut butter chips (optional) (you will need to buy vegan chips to prepare truly dairy-free)

Colored sugar (optional)

1. Grease a 9 by 13-inch baking pan. Premeasure the marshmallows, cereal, and chips before you move ahead to step 2. You will need to work quickly so that the mixture does not set before you have mixed all the ingredients.

2. Melt the butter in a medium-size saucepan over low heat and add the marshmallows, stirring constantly until the marshmallows have melted.

3. Remove from the heat and gradually add the cereal, quickly stirring well to coat. Stir in the peanut butter chips before the mixture hardens, then pour into the prepared pan. Use a rubber spatula or a small square of waxed paper that has been sprayed with cooking spray to pat the mixture into the pan and smooth it out. Sprinkle with colored sugar, if using, and allow to cool before cutting.

IN A SENTENCE

Making crowd-pleasing recipes like these, you should never hesitate to host or attend any social function, even on a gluten-free diet.

HALF-YEAR MILESTONE

Over the past six months, you have learned much about adapting to your new gluten-free life. Having first gained a solid understanding of the dynamics of celiac disease, you have been able to concentrate in recent months on learning to face many social situations confidently. You can now look ahead to learning even more tips to hone your gluten-free life skills. You have learned:

○ How to have a clean, organized, and largely gluten-free kitchen and shop with confidence

○ How to handle sticky situations such as dating and college life

○ How to safely eat out at restaurants and consume gluten-free alcohols

○ How to find support from others who are living gluten-free and share your information with people who may benefit from knowing about CD

○ About the connection between celiac disease and infertility, and what to do if you have infertility or pregnancy complications

○ Recipes and tips for gluten-free entertaining

Your Child and Celiac Disease

Testing Your Child for Celiac Disease

If you or a member of your immediate family has been diagnosed with celiac disease, it is natural that you would have concerns about whether to test your children. Since celiac disease is a hereditary condition that arises in 1 out of every 22 people with CD positive first-degree relatives and 1 out of every 39 second-degree relatives, a positive diagnosis in a member of your family may drive you to have others tested as well, even if they are asymptomatic.[1]

Many pediatricians regularly screen for celiac disease in all of their patients with celiac family members. Such screenings should occur every two to three years beginning at the age of two, even if the children don't seem to have symptoms. In addition, children with Down syndrome, diabetes, irritable bowel syndrome, or any autoimmune diseases should also be screened. My children's pediatrician, Dr. Monique Burke, also urges all

---

1. A. Fasano et al., "A Multi-Center Study on the Sero-Prevalence of Celiac Disease in the United States among Both at Risk and Not at Risk Groups," *Archives of Internal Medicine* 163 (February 2003): 286–92.

parents of children with celiac-affected relatives to be more aware of possible subtle manifestations of celiac disease and to bring these conditions to her attention so that early diagnosis is possible. Some of the changes she reports seeing most often include a change in bowel habits, eating/nutritional changes, and even changes in a child's behavior in conjunction with medical abnormalities.

Since serological screening can be traumatic for children, I elect to have my asymptomatic children only tested at regular intervals when other blood work is necessary. For my son, I had him tested at his second birthday and upon the start of kindergarten; my daughter is three and she has been tested once so far. Certainly, if my children manifested any overt and otherwise unexplained symptoms that could be indicative of celiac disease, I would not hesitate to request laboratory studies at any time.[2] Dr. Burke also recommends more frequent testing if there is any change in family medical history, a change in the patient's own medical history, or if other laboratory studies are needed on a regular basis for other conditions such as Down syndrome. In her general pediatric practice, she finds that she typically has cause to screen at least one pediatric patient weekly for celiac disease.

Although these serological studies are excellent screening tools, they are frequently less reliable in young children. Therefore, both parents and physicians need to be vigilant in watching for changes in the child's health and in repeating screenings if the child falls into any high-risk category. Do not simply put your children on a gluten-free diet without testing, though, as accurate testing to confirm celiac disease will be difficult or impossible if the child is already on a gluten-free diet.

If serological testing is negative but the child nonetheless manifests suspicious symptoms, your pediatrician may at that point recommend endoscopic testing or a referral to a pediatric gastroenterologist. If testing is ultimately negative but your child is still not well, at that point, trying a gluten-free diet is certainly worth the effort. Gluten intolerance or even undiagnosed celiac disease may still be the root cause and a gluten-free diet may just be the key to your child's good health.

---

2. D. Hill et al., "Clinical Guideline: Guideline for the Diagnosis and Treatment of Celiac Disease in Children: Recommendations of the North American Society for Pediatric Gastroenterology, Hepatatology and Nutrition," *Journal of Pediatric Gastroenterology and Nutrition* 40, no. 1 (January 2005): 1–19.

Introducing Gluten to Your Child's Diet

Another area of concern for celiac parents is at what age gluten should be introduced into their infants' diets. Recent research on when to introduce gluten seems to suggest that between four and six months of age is the optimum time,[3] although other long-term studies that are underway may yield different results. Still other studies seem to indicate that breast-feeding may offer protection against developing celiac disease.[4] Due to the newness of these studies, it is unclear whether or not breast-feeding merely delays the onset of symptoms or permanently protects against the disease. However, several studies have confirmed that gradually introducing gluten into infants' diets while they are still being breast-fed does reduce the risk of developing celiac disease in early childhood.[5] In fact, exclusively breast-fed children are reported to be significantly less likely to report failure to thrive and short stature.[6]

Parents with celiac in the family have good cause to closely monitor and test their children since celiac disease is hereditary. More and more pediatricians are recommending regular screening for even asymptomatic patients with celiac family members. Early detection, before the disease can have more severe and long-lasting adverse effects, is key to limiting the damage it can cause to developing children.

IN A SENTENCE

> *As celiac disease is hereditary, monitoring subtle health changes in your children, having regular serological testing, and maintaining close contact with your children's pediatrician can minimize the risk that undetected celiac disease could be harming your youngsters.*

3. Stephano Guandalini, MD, "Celiac Disease Does Not Cause Infertility in the U.S. or Does It?" *Impact* 8, no. 1 (Winter 2008): 1–2; Jill M. Norris et al., "Risk of Celiac Disease Autoimmunity and Timing of Gluten Introduction in the Diet of Infants at Increased Risk of Disease," *Journal of the American Medical Association* 293, no. 19 (May 18, 2005): 2343–51.

4. A. K. Akobeng et al., "Effect of Breast Feeding on Risk of Cœliac Disease: A Systematic Review and Meta-Analysis Of Observational Studies," *Archives of Disease in Childhood* 91 (2006): 39–43.

5. Anneli Ivarsson et al., "Breast-Feeding Protects against Celiac Disease," *American Journal of Clinical Nutrition* 75, no. 5 (May 2002): 914–21.

6. Michael A. d'Amico et al., "Presentation of Pediatric Celiac Disease in the United States: Prominent Effect of Breastfeeding," *Clinical Pediatrics* 44, no. 3 (2005): 249–58.

A Pediatrician's Perspective: Dr. Monique Burke[7]

As a general pediatrician, it is my role to monitor the growth and development of all of my patients. Each visit to the pediatrician focuses on growth charts and developmental milestones. These visits are also filled with advice for the coming months. Many times, this advice pertains to car seats, safe play places, and sleep habits. Nutrition is also an important topic of conversation. Pediatricians generally agree that breast-feeding is best for infants, but when and how to introduce solid foods is a hot topic of recent research. It is during this time that infants/children with celiac disease may begin to manifest symptoms.

Celiac disease is not new to the pediatric radar. The classic presentation was thought to occur in infancy and result in a failure to thrive. These infants grow well during the first months when they are exclusively breast/formula fed. After the introduction of solid foods, between four and six months, their growth starts to fall off the growth chart. A change in the growth curve is a red flag for pediatricians. If the growth continues to slow, it is frequently necessary for the physician to investigate the cause. This examination typically involves blood work and urine collection.

Celiac disease is frequently on the differential diagnosis for infants and children with poor growth and/or gastrointestinal symptoms. These symptoms may present as chronic diarrhea, abdominal distention, irritability, vomiting, or constipation. If any infant/child demonstrates the above symptoms for a prolonged period of time, it is important to discuss these manifestations with your pediatrician. Accurate diagnosis and treatment require timely recognition of warning symptoms. Initial screening tests (such as blood work) may be ordered by your physician. If screening tests are positive or if there remains a high level of suspicion after negative testing, a referral to a pediatric gastroenterologist may be in order.

---

7. Monique Soileau-Burke, MD, FAAP, is in private pediatric practice in Catonsville, Maryland. She is a graduate of Tulane Medical School in New Orleans, Louisiana, and did her pediatric residency training at the Johns Hopkins School of Medicine in Baltimore, Maryland.

living

Parenting a Child with Celiac Disease

ANGIE AND Cade's story captures the feeling of being overwhelmed but beginning to look ahead, grateful that celiac disease is the diagnosis. As Angie reminds herself and us, we must all be thankful that CD can be managed with diet instead of lifelong medications, treatments, and surgeries.

◇ ◇ ◇

Angie Dabbs's Story

The summer of 2007 started as most summers do, with fun-filled days outdoors, vacation plans at the beach, and a carefree spirit. It promised to be an especially exciting summer and one full of anticipation: our daughter was gearing up for kindergarten in the fall, our son was looking forward to starting preschool, and we were all eagerly awaiting the birth of our third child that coming September. But, our excited spirit quickly gave way to confusion and despair when our son, Cade, then two and a half, was diagnosed as celiac. The diagnosis would prove to be a journey for our family: a test of our strength, an introduction to the world of natural food markets (and an accompanying challenge to our frugality), a fierce sense of advocacy for our son and his condition, and, ultimately, newfound hope and the realization that celiac disease is manageable.

Unlike most celiac patients who suffer through countless misdiagnoses and long bouts of intestinal distress, Cade's symptoms were seemingly sudden, and his diagnosis was relatively swift. For this, we were grateful. The diagnosis was, nonetheless, harrowing for our family.

Cade initially developed a fairly typical stomach virus, but after ten days of uncharacteristic irritability, frequent diarrhea, and a low-grade fever, his pediatrician started focusing on his virus more aggressively. Initial blood work indicated a low level of protein in his body, and the levels continued to drop dangerously low. In a matter of days, our lives seemed to be spiraling out of control. My husband and I ended up taking Cade to the emergency room, and from there, Cade was transported via ambulance to Children's Hospital in Washington, D.C., where we spent three long days and nights.

Getting to a Diagnosis

The possible diagnoses were frightening. Although the doctors were cautious to not speculate, it was difficult for us to control our wandering minds. Was it cancer? Would Cade die? How could our innocent, energetic, strawberry-blond-haired, blue-eyed, charming little guy be so sick? It would be more than twenty-four hours before we received an answer.

In the meantime, Cade continued to swell. Although we never weighed him while he was in the hospital, he appeared significantly heavier. His sweet little eyes were almost swollen shut, his lean frame was bloated, and he was inconsolable most of the time. It broke my heart to see him like that, and my husband and I felt helpless.

Reaching a diagnosis was not without invasive—but necessary—testing. In addition to multiple blood draws, Cade underwent an endoscopy and sigmoidoscopy. Watching our little son be wheeled away on a gurney as he sobbed, "Daddy!" was probably the most heart-wrenching experience my husband and I have had as parents. And the wait for the results seemed to last an eternity.

As the specialists began mentioning celiac disease, we were shocked. We knew very little about the disease, and we weren't aware of a family history of it. Considering the prognoses that bombarded our minds over the preceding days, though, we tried to focus on feeling optimistic and relieved. We promised ourselves that we would need to be very grateful if the celiac diagnosis was confirmed.

In the end, we were sent home with our sweet little boy and a firm diagnosis of celiac disease. As the doctors explained to us, the disease often emerges as a result of an injury, severe stress, trauma, or—in Cade's case—an illness. We went on to learn that Cade had had this genetic disease since birth even though he was asymptomatic until he contracted that virus. Now confused and distraught, our carefree spirit during the start of the summer seemed like a distant memory. Our entire focus was on Cade. I was on a mission to learn everything I could about this disease, and I felt a tremendous sense of urgency to do so.

I remember telling my colleague in those first days that I didn't feel as if I'd had enough time to process the diagnosis, and that the lack of processing felt unnatural to me. He said pointedly, "Sometimes it's best not to process." Retrospectively, he was probably right. As quickly as the situation seemed to unravel, we had to pick up the pieces and forge ahead, and I'm not sure that "processing" the diagnosis would have been healthy or helpful. Forging ahead was difficult, though, especially in the first weeks.

Our Learning Curve

The first few times I went grocery shopping were devastating. I remember standing in the aisles, crying, trying to master label-reading with my CliffNotes in hand. Through tears, I read label after label and became more discouraged with each one. I pictured the future and the countless restrictions Cade would face. I wondered how I would master all that I needed to know to keep him safe and healthy. I was completely overwhelmed, and the emotion I felt then is still so potent now. This was the first time as a parent that I'd experienced anything like this. But I had to remind myself that I was grateful for the celiac diagnosis.

We went to the beach just two weeks after Cade's diagnosis, for our annual family trip. The vacation was different in several respects and full of new learnings. We packed the vast majority of our food—mostly gluten-free—and cooked almost all of our meals in the kitchen of the condo. We discovered the difficulty and uncertainty of grabbing a snack from an eatery while out on the boardwalk. We continued exposing our son to his new foods and explaining why his favorites (oatmeal, Cheerios, whole wheat bread) went away. But, most significantly, we realized a strong sense of gratitude for being together—and healthy—that we probably didn't acknowledge in the years prior to Cade's diagnosis. And, after just a couple of weeks, we were all adapting. So, hope was definitely in order.

The learning curve was significant in the beginning, and we made lots of mistakes. I remember buying a crispy rice–type cereal, thinking, "Cade can eat rice, so this will be fine." Later, after rechecking the ingredients, I remembered that malt was a taboo ingredient, and the brand I had purchased was therefore off-limits. We didn't fully understand the implications of cross-contamination issues in the beginning, so we made some mistakes in that area, too. But we became more knowledgeable as time went on, and we learned to be patient with ourselves as we tried to wrap our minds around the disease and the lifestyle change.

As we move through the months since Cade's diagnosis, the journey continues. While we haven't mastered the disease (Does anyone ever master it?), we have come a long way. I still visit the road of despair every now and then. Sometimes it's difficult to not feel sorry for Cade, especially when he's attending a birthday party or preschool function laden with gluten-filled foods. But, I try to think about my vow to be grateful, and I exit to the road of optimism, which is where Cade needs me to be.

It Does Get Easier

Today, label-reading is second nature for me, the aisles in the natural food markets are ingrained in my brain, and I'm a member of the unofficially chartered club of moms who have children with celiac disease, food allergies, and other related concerns. My husband and I have discovered tremendous resources devoted to celiac disease, and we continue to discover more. Our neighborhood grocery store chains are beginning to carry more and more gluten-free foods, making it easier and more affordable to shop. Cade has adapted beautifully to his gluten-free diet and accepts that he has a "special tummy," a term coined by a wonderful friend whose daughter has food allergies. And perhaps the sweetest outcome of all, Cade and I have developed a special bond through baking together. We both love our weekly baking sessions, where we make a mess, nibble on ingredients, and enjoy the concoctions we create together. Cade is always excited to share his baked goods with his daddy and big sister, and he is quick to say, "When the baby gets bigger, he can eat this, too!"

I've learned that celiac disease is a drastic lifestyle change. It requires adherence to a specialized diet and monitoring by a savvy gastroenterologist. And, for children, it means an early lesson in being different. But, I've also learned that celiac disease is not a death sentence. It is manageable today, and it will become even more manageable in the future as the medical community uncovers new advances; as stores carry and vendors develop more gluten-free products; and as more of our neighbors, friends, and family members are diagnosed.

I've learned a lot about myself since Cade's diagnosis, and my perspective on life has certainly broadened. This has probably aided me in the many roles I have in life, including that of advocate for my son. In a paradoxical sort of way, I have Cade's diagnosis to thank for my generally more optimistic way of viewing things. After all, there is much about which to be optimistic. And Cade—with his special tummy and lovable demeanor—is proof!

◇ ◇ ◇

IN A SENTENCE

Any parent who has suffered with and for their sick child understands the true nature of feeling "grateful" for a celiac diagnosis; Angie Dabbs's determination to help her child live happily and healthily by simply controlling his diet is a fantastic model for us all.

learning

Kids' Birthday Parties

I F I had to pick the one question I am asked most from my consulting clients, it is "How can I help my child with celiac feel 'normal'?" Birthday parties are a big part of this answer. I am devoting nearly an entire chapter to kids' gluten-free birthday parties because they are *that* important.

The first thing to remember with regard to children's birthdays is that your children will attend far more birthday parties for other children than they will have parties of their own. Therefore, you must create a plan for how to handle these parties and still maintain your sanity! I won't tell you that it isn't a lot of work, but the payoffs are enormous and there are some easy tips to making the whole experience a lot less time-consuming for you.

School Parties

Many children's parties take place at school. Different schools and age groups approach birthday parties in different ways, but the traditional bring-cupcakes-to-school birthday is still fairly widespread. Recently, I have encountered a lot of schools that have instituted policies banning homemade goodies for these parties because of food allergies. They require store-bought treats with clear food labels indicating ingredients. This policy presumes that bakeries at local grocers are on the ball enough to print all the ingredients and to prevent cross-contamination in their kitchens. These policies are flawed in other ways as well, including the fact that the selected treats almost certainly contain gluten, and they discourage family participation in the kitchen to prepare and decorate the treats (something I advocate for!). Although I believe such policies are well intentioned and have more than likely been instituted in response to complaints, incidents, and lawsuits over food allergies, these policies are overly broad and reactionary. It is a shame that the result of these actions is to actually make things *worse* for people with food allergies or CD, because they remove parental controls and participation!

There are plenty of reasons to complain about rules such as these when you have a child with celiac disease. The best response though is to be proactive when you are considering what school your child will attend or when you prepare for your child's first school year. Question what the school policy is on birthday parties and other events where parents can bring in goodies *before* your child begins school there. You will have a much easier time getting information before the first day of school begins and chaos breaks out! If you are dissatisfied with the answer (such as that the school observes a policy like the one discussed above), then make an appointment to speak with the principal to discuss your concerns. Obviously, if there is a gluten-free bakery in your area, bringing in those desserts with food labels solves the problem easily, but if not, you need to approach the issue from a different angle.

Making the Argument for Homemade Goodies at School Parties

○ The most persuasive argument in this type of case is made when you are calm, rational, and kind.

○ Clearly explain your child's food restrictions, supplementing with information from your physician, if necessary.

○ Propose that you be permitted to bring your own homemade goodies for your child and for the class on your child's birthday.

○ Offer to bring in clear ingredient lists as well, thereby rendering your food as information-friendly as store-bought items.

continued

○ Ask if there are any other children in your child's class who have food allergies—seek out these parents to come up with a plan together.

○ Propose that you be permitted to draw up a flier for the school to send home with all the children in that class, explaining the recipe and ingredients of the treat(s) you intend to bring before the date of your child's party and instructing parents to send an alternative treat with their own child if there is an ingredient to which their child has an allergy.

○ For other children's parties, ask if you may send in a dozen gluten-free cupcakes and have them stored in the freezer of the teacher's lounge or cafeteria—whichever is more convenient for the teacher to access for your child.

○ Or, ask that you be informed in advance of any other child's birthday celebration in the class, so that you can send in an alternative treat for your child that day.

○ Move up the hierarchy of authority at the school until you achieve an adequate solution.

○ If you cannot reach a resolution, consider changing schools and finding another school with more flexibility and responsiveness to your child's needs.

○ As a last resort, contact local news media to alert them to the problem in the school. Your child is not and will not be the only one to face the same problem due to food allergies and intolerances.

It is imperative that celiac children be able to participate in special events like these to gain the self-confidence and acceptance from other students necessary to foster their personal growth in these formative years. If your child's school is not supportive of these efforts and will not work with you to assure that your child have positive social experiences despite food restrictions, you should either move up the ladder to speak with the school superintendent or move your child to another school if possible. We have all learned through our own personal experiences that the squeaky wheel gets the grease: people seem to be most squeaky (and thereby most successful) when the issue pertains to their children. You will be successful if you are creative, flexible, and nonthreatening when dealing with the school authorities. They should want to help your child, so help them to help you.

Attending Birthday Parties

When it comes to attending parties away from school, the problem is often much more easily solved. An RSVP is necessary, so when you do so, discuss with the other parent what the best option is to provide a treat for your child without disrupting or imposing on the host. Other parents will respect your child's needs when you make it clear to them and will not begrudge you or your child if you make it easy on them or make treats to share with all the children. You make the treat; you bring the treat; you clearly but politely explain to the host that this is the only treat your child may eat; you make sure your child knows which treat is his or hers; you show appropriate gratitude for the graciousness of the host; your child gets invited back again.

Your Child's Party

Your child's own birthday party should be the time when he or she feels special and totally normal. Your focus should be on offering yummy foods and treats that all guests will enjoy together (and that, of course, will all be gluten-free). There should be no discussion of the fact that the food is gluten-free, unless another parent comes to you to discuss a food allergy. If you host the party at your house, the plan is simple. If you host the party elsewhere, you just have to be sure before you book the party that the facility is amenable to you bringing in your own cake and other food, if necessary. This agreement should be secured in writing so there is no misunderstanding on party day.

As for the menu, your child's own tastes and age to a certain extent will dictate what you provide. Whatever your theme, you can devise a plan for foods that will complement the party and will be enjoyed by everyone in attendance. The next section, beginning on page 175, features several very kid-friendly recipes ideal for birthday parties. (Be sure to try them in advance of any party so that you are sure you can make enough, and that your child really likes them.)

Party Possiblities

Listed below are several party ideas; think outside the box and be creative. Having to think gluten-free could be the catalyst you need to create the perfect party!

- Let the attendees decorate their cookies or cupcakes—arm all the children with colored sugar and gluten-free tubes of store-bought icing.
- Have a taco-making party with all the fixin's.

○ Hide a gummy bear inside your gluten-free cake batter and have a game to see which guest finds the gummy bear in his or her piece of cake! (Haribo Gummi Bears are gluten-free.)

○ Throw an ice-cream sundae party with gluten-free toppings.

○ Make crispy rice treats cut out in different shapes to match your theme, frost them, and use them as edible decorations (be sure to use gluten-free crispy rice cereal).

○ Include a piñata filled with gluten-free candy, plus temporary tattoos, rubber balls, and other nonedible favors.

○ Give a pirate party with gluten-free fish sticks and homemade gluten-free hush puppies.

○ Have the kids make s'mores, using gluten-free graham crackers.

○ Take a group to the movies and treat everyone to popcorn.

○ Take a small group to a restaurant that offers a gluten-free dessert for everyone to share.

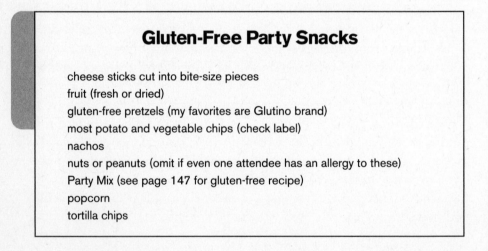

Gluten-Free Party Snacks

cheese sticks cut into bite-size pieces

fruit (fresh or dried)

gluten-free pretzels (my favorites are Glutino brand)

most potato and vegetable chips (check label)

nachos

nuts or peanuts (omit if even one attendee has an allergy to these)

Party Mix (see page 147 for gluten-free recipe)

popcorn

tortilla chips

IN A SENTENCE

Birthday parties—ones you host, ones at school, and those at your child's friends' homes—are not-to-be-missed formative affairs that, with a little gluten-free planning on your part, can help your child feel "normal" (or "special," depending on whose party it is).

living

Gluten-Free Recipes
Perfect for Kids and Parties

NO ONE likes to attend a party and have to sit on the side-lines when the cake and other edible yummies are brought out. These recipes for such party staples as pizza, cheese sticks, and cakes (including the frosting) allow everyone attending to indulge, and even work in some added nutrition in the process . . . providing yet another reason to celebrate!

Gluten-Free Fish Sticks

COMMERCIALLY AVAILABLE gluten-free fish sticks are carried in many organic markets and are pretty tasty—one brand is Ian's (they also have non-gluten-free fish sticks, so be sure to buy the right package)—but they can be rather expensive, especially if you are trying to feed a party of hungry junior pirates! I recommend making a large batch with this recipe (multiply by three or four, depending on the size of your party) and using a mild marinara or pasta sauce for dipping. I either buy a premade sauce with lots of pureed vegetables inside or make it myself and load it with extra pureed vegetables. It's just about the only way my kids will gladly eat their veggies.

Makes 12 to 15 fish sticks

Olive oil, for oiling skillet

4 fillets of white fish, such as tilapia or halibut

1 1/2 cups Nearly Normal All-Purpose Flour (page 48)

2 eggs, beaten

1/2 cup Konriko Fish Fry*

1 cup gluten-free bread crumbs (make your own or use such brands as Hol-Grain Brown Rice Bread Crumbs)

1. Preheat the oven to 450°F. Oil a large skillet with olive oil, and grease a cookie sheet.

2. Prepare three bowls long enough to fit your longest fish stick. The first bowl should have the Nearly Normal All-Purpose Flour; the second, the beaten eggs; the third, the fish fry mixture stirred with the bread crumbs.

3. Cut fish into fish stick–size strips and clean them. Dredge in Nearly Normal All-Purpose Flour. Next, dip into the beaten eggs. Finally, dredge in the fish fry mixture.

4. Flash-fry the dipped fish sticks in the prepared skillet for approximately 30 seconds—1 minute per side. Lay each flash-fried stick onto the prepared cookie sheet. Bake in the preheated oven for 10 minutes, turn and bake for 3 to 5 more minutes, or until the sides are crispy and light brown and the fish is flaky inside.

---

*You may prepare your own fish fry mixture, by combining the following:

1/2 cup gluten-free bread crumbs

1/4 cup grated Parmesan cheese (optional)

1 tablespoon onion powder

1 teaspoon garlic salt

1 teaspoon sea salt

1/2 teaspoon black pepper

1/2 teaspoon red pepper or cayenne (if you want it spicy; optional)

Pizza

THIS RECIPE makes an amazingly real pizza crust! It rises and produces a wonderfully chewy crust that is perfect for sharing. Top with whatever ingredients you and your child like best, but make sure you make enough for the rest of the party! This dough recipe makes one, approximately 14-inch, crust.

$1^1/2$ cups Nearly Normal All-Purpose Flour (page 48)

3 tablespoons dry milk powder

$1/4$ teaspoon dried oregano

Pinch or two of garlic powder

$1/2$ teaspoon salt

$2^1/2$ teaspoons rapid-rise yeast (approximately one $1/4$-ounce packet)

2 egg whites

2 tablespoons olive oil

$1/2$ teaspoon apple cider vinegar

$3/4$ cup warm water

1. Preheat the oven to 375°F. Oil a pizza pan or baking stone reserved for gluten-free cooking only.

2. Blend the dry ingredients in a large bowl. Combine the wet ingredients in another bowl, reserving some of the water, and add to the dry ingredients. Mix with an electric mixer on low. Add the Nearly Normal All-Purpose Flour, and continue beating. Add more water as needed to get a firm, sticky dough that can still be spread. Beat at high speed for 3 minutes once the flour has been added.

3. Spoon the dough onto the prepared pan. Spread into a 14-inch circle, using a flat spoon or your oiled hands. Raise the edges so the topping won't fall off. Let rise for about 10 minutes and then bake for about 15 minutes. The baking time will vary, depending on your pan.

4. Spread with your desired toppings and cook an additional 20 minutes, or until the cheese is bubbly. If you add vegetable toppings, I find they taste best if you sauté them in olive oil before adding them to the crust.

Baked Cheese Sticks

WHAT KID (or adult, for that matter) wouldn't love to have ooey-gooey, hot cheese sticks dipped in yummy marinara sauce? If you use reduced-fat cheese sticks and puree loads of healthy veggies to add to any gluten-free commercially sold red sauce, the kids will never even know that this dish is full of vitamins and minerals!

1/2 cup canola oil, for frying

1/3 cup Nearly Normal All-Purpose Flour (page 48)

1 egg, mixed

1 tablespoon skim milk

1/2 cup Hol-Grain Chicken Coating Mix*

8 reduced-fat mozzarella sticks or string cheese

1 cup marinara sauce

1. Heat the canola oil in an electric skillet to 375° to 400°F, or in a large stove-top skillet over medium-high heat.

2. Pour the Nearly Normal All-Purpose Flour into a small bowl. Whisk the egg and milk in a second small bowl. In a third bowl, place the mixed crumb coating.

3. Roll each cheese stick in the gluten-free flour, then in the egg mixture, then in the crumb coating, covering all sides and ends of the sticks. Then repeat in the egg, then crumb coating.

4. Carefully place the coated sticks into the hot oil and cook for approximately 2 minutes, then turn to cook the other side. The sticks should be a crisp brown color, but not burned, and the cheese may be melting from cracks in the coating. Lay the sticks onto a cookie sheet and place into the warm oven if you are not serving immediately, otherwise, transfer the sticks to high-quality paper towels to absorb the oil before serving.

5. Serve warm with a small bowl of marinara sauce on the side, for dipping.

---

* If you would prefer to make your own bread crumb coating, use the following recipe:

1/2 cup gluten-free dried bread crumbs or corn flake crumbs

1/4 teaspoon red pepper

1/4 teaspoon black pepper

1/4 teaspoon garlic powder

1/4 teaspoon sea salt

1/2 teaspoon dried parsley

1/8 teaspoon chile powder

Birthday Cake

WHAT BIRTHDAY party (or any kind of party, for that matter!) is complete without a delicious, indulgent, decorated cake? I have devised so many recipes now for clients with all kinds of food allergies that I have tried endless substitutions and alternatives. I have noted several below and in the text box as well. I have provided recipes for a yellow cake and a chocolate cake so that the honoree may choose his or her favorite for that special day. These cakes rise nicely and do not have huge cave-ins, as do so many other gluten-free cakes. They are so moist and flavorful, you will want to find other occasions to make these fun recipes!

Yellow Cake

3 cups Nearly Normal All-Purpose Flour (page 48)

1 tablespoon gluten-free baking powder

1 teaspoon baking soda

1/4 teaspoon salt

1 1/2 cups sugar

1/4 cup dry buttermilk powder, or 1 1/2 teaspoons unflavored gelatin to make a nondairy cake

2 eggs, or for an egg-free cake use the equivalent of egg substitute such as Ener-G brand

1/2 cup vanilla dairy or soy yogurt or canola oil

2 teaspoons gluten-free vanilla extract

1 3/4 cups plain or vanilla-flavor milk (see text box for nondairy milk alternatives)

Chocolate Cake

3 cups Nearly Normal All-Purpose Flour (page 48)

1 tablespoon gluten-free baking powder

1 teaspoon baking soda

1/4 teaspoon salt

1 1/2 cups sugar

1/4 cup dry buttermilk powder, or 1 1/2 teaspoons unflavored gelatin to make a nondairy cake

2 eggs, or for an egg-free cake use the equivalent of egg substitute such as Ener-G brand

1/2 cup vanilla dairy or soy yogurt or canola oil

2 teaspoons gluten-free vanilla extract

2 cups chocolate milk (see text box for nondairy milk alternatives)

1/4 cup unsweetened cocoa powder

1. Preheat the oven to 300°F if convection (recommended) or 325°F if nonconvection. Prepare a 9 by 13-inch pan or two 9-inch round pans by lightly coating with cooking oil and dusting with corn- or potato starch. Alternatively, you may melt 2 tablespoons of shortening into the bottom of the pan(s) and turn each pan so that the entire bottom and lower sides are coated. Put the pan(s) into the freezer for 15 minutes, then remove and set aside.

2. Whisk the dry ingredients together in a large bowl. Stir the egg and yogurt together in a second, small bowl, then add to the dry ingredients and stir. Add the milk slowly while beating the entire mixture. Beat until smooth, then beat for an additional 1 to 2 minutes, until the batter is light.

3. Pour into prepared cake pan(s) and bake for 35 to 45 minutes, depending on the pan size and whether you are using the convection setting. The cake should have a lightly browned crown and a cake tester inserted into the middle of the pan should test cleanly.

4. Resist the temptation to open the oven door to check on the cake. Every time the door is opened, the oven temperature fluctuates and can cause shrinkage or caving in. Use your oven light to peek at your cake, opening the door only when you truly think the cake might be done. When the cake tests done, turn the oven off but leave the cake in the oven with the door open. This will allow a more gradual cooling of the cake and also cause less contraction.

5. When totally cooled, remove gently from the pan(s) and frost with your favorite frosting.

Nondairy Milk Alternatives in Baking

Think outside the carton. Of course, you can always use gluten-free rice or soy milk as a substitute, but why not look for more flavorful and nutritious options? Try substitutes such as Bolthouse Farms "Perfectly Protein" Vanilla Chai Tea with Soy Protein—a wonderful substitute for milk in recipes like cakes. This drink is a thick soy milk and green tea mixture with natural fruit juice sweeteners and added vitamins and minerals.

Another option is vanilla- or chocolate-flavor Almond Breeze. This dairy-free, casein-free milk alternative is made from almonds, water, and cane juice and has added vitamins and minerals.

Tofutti brand now has gluten- and milk-free cream cheese and sour cream, so feel free to use these to open up new options for your dairy-free baking!

Gluten-Free Frosting Options

Banana Frosting

$1/2$ cup mashed bananas (approximately 2 bananas)

2 teaspoons fresh lemon juice, or $1/4$ scant teaspoon True Lemon plus
   2 teaspoons water

$1/2$ cup butter or nondairy alternative

$31/2$–4 cups confectioners' sugar

1 teaspoon gluten-free vanilla extract

1. In a small bowl, mix the mashed bananas and lemon juice. Set aside.

2. In another bowl, cream the butter and sugar with an electric mixer until light and fluffy. Add the mashed banana mixture and vanilla, blending until well mixed. If you are making a layer cake, try laying additional sliced bananas on top of the frosting in the layer between the cakes—it makes a pretty and tasty center for a yellow or chocolate cake.

Cream Cheese Frosting

8 ounces dairy or soy cream cheese, room temperature

$1/2$ cup butter or nondairy alternative

2 cups confectioners' sugar

1 teaspoon gluten-free vanilla extract

1 cup finely chopped pecans (optional)

1. Combine the cream cheese and butter in a bowl, beating with an electric mixer until smooth.

2. Add the confectioners' sugar and vanilla, continuing to beat until the frosting is light and fluffy. Stir in the nuts at this point, if using.

White Frosting (Base)

¼ cup milk (see text box for nondairy milk alternatives)

½ cup butter or nondairy alternative, softened

2½ cups confectioners' sugar

1½ teaspoons gluten-free vanilla extract

1. Cream the milk and butter together in a bowl with an electric mixer. Add half of the sugar, beating well to combine, then add the remaining ingredients, beating for several minutes until light and fluffy.

Chocolate Frosting

Use the white frosting base recipe and add ½ cup of unsweetened cocoa powder with the remaining ingredients.

Mocha Frosting

Use the white frosting base recipe, but substitute cold coffee, cappuccino, or espresso for the milk. Add ¼ cup unsweetened cocoa powder as well, when adding the remaining ingredients.

ABOUT PREMADE FROSTING

Several brands of ready-made frostings are already gluten-free! So if you lack the time or inclination, you can always run to your local grocer. Remember to always check labels or Web sites for current product information, but the brand that seems to have the most gluten-free choices as of 2008 is Pillsbury.

IN A SENTENCE

You can throw a gluten-free party with scrumptious eats that will be talked about long after the party itself, and since you won't even have to divulge that the foods were gluten-free, every get-together you host can be a bit of a surprise party!

Handling the Holidays

HOLIDAYS FOR anyone are fraught with a mixture of eager anticipation, happy exhaustion, and agonizing overplanning. Add celiac disease to the mix and things just get more complicated, but you don't have to feel overwhelmed.

So how does one with food restrictions cope in our food-saturated society, particularly at the holidays? There is no one-size-fits-all answer to such a loaded question, but try this one out: pretend you're just like everyone else. That's right—share an amazing Thanksgiving spread with your friends and family, break out the challah, bake holiday cookies as gifts, and deal with the added pounds later . . . just like everyone else! I don't mean to say you should eat things that are forbidden to you, but I do mean that you should make your favorite foods safe for your diet while still being delicious for you and your whole family.

One of the easiest ways to make the modifications necessary to put this theory into action is to host your own holiday parties. Just like when you are entertaining for fun at other times of the year, volunteer to have your guests enjoy the holidays in your home. This way, you can control not only the recipe content but any cross-contamination fears. You need not be forever saddled with all future family seders or Christmas dinners but, particularly in the beginning, you will always feel more comfortable on your own turf. Once your family tastes the delicious recipes you offer, they will want to make them, too, and future family events will be much easier to navigate. Gluten-free foods and their preparation is an education for everyone whose lives touch yours, so expect a lot of questions and be ready to answer them with savory alternatives to wheat-based traditional favorites.

◇ ◇ ◇

A Whole New Gluten-Free Approach to the Holidays: Chrissy Andrews's Story

Since my diagnosis one year ago, my older sister and our mother have also been diagnosed with celiac disease. As a family, we have experienced a culinary 180-degree turn and our kitchen now has two separate sections: one we call "gluten-free" and one called "gluten-full." We distinguish between the gluten-free and gluten-full condiments, for example, and have separate bins for different items.

There are six of us in my family: three of us eat gluten-free and three don't. However, all of us have worked hard to ensure that all the gluten-free food stays uncontaminated and readily available, and we all try to work together to form new solutions that are good for everyone. For celebrations, there is always a gluten-free option if not an entirely gluten-free meal (desserts included, of course!). We have a family meal almost every night and have found that we are all eating healthier foods, less preservatives, and more home-cooked meals.

That said, eating gluten-free makes every social situation different from how it used to be. When it is just our immediate family at the house, it is easier—there are no worries of contamination or concern over bland and incomplete meals. However, this protected home environment is not always possible. I never realized how many special occasions center on food! Holidays are also complicated because they usually rotate between families hosting the event and there are many traditional meals for each holiday. While trying not to change these traditions or take away from anyone else's enjoyment, we have tried to come up with gluten-free solutions. For example, the cake for my parent's twenty-fifth wedding anniversary party was gluten-free. We decided not to mention it until everyone already ate it, and the cake was complimented heavily before anyone even knew. Most people didn't even know it was possible to make a gluten-free cake!

For Thanksgiving (my personal favorite holiday) this first year after my diagnosis, my family decided to take a new approach and meet at a cabin in the Pennsylvania mountains for a long weekend. We cooked a delicious gluten-free meal, just the six of us, and visited relatives in the following days surrounding Thanksgiving. It was a great solution for us this year as we did not feel like an imposition on any extended family (six people and three with special dietary needs is a lot to throw on any one family), but we still enjoyed great food and got to visit with relatives during the holiday.

My family offered to host Christmas dinner for the first time ever this past year. Coming up with the menu, we tried to incorporate the traditional dishes that are usually served at my grandparent's house, with some options for us. Also, cooking the food in our own kitchen ensured that we could be positive our food would be free of contamination issues or hidden gluten. We cooked a turkey with stuffing on the side and not inside it and served baked potatoes and vegetables. The meal definitely had more healthy options than our past Christmas dinners had, but we made it a point to keep favorite dishes and a variety of desserts so there was something for everyone. We had no complaints and many compliments about the food!

There have been so many changes in our family in the last year related to gluten-free living: new food products, new kitchen appliances, new kitchen organization, new meals cooked, a refocus on overall health (including yoga). There is no way we can host every event or holiday, but we can always bring a gluten-free dish to share. I am sure we will continue to adjust our strategies to make it the most comfortable situation possible. However, I think the biggest change is how close our family has become. No piece of bread would ever be worth changing that.

◇ ◇ ◇

IN A SENTENCE

Particularly in the beginning, you'll find it's easiest to host a holiday meal yourself so you have control over the food; being a guest is easy if you bring along a modified version of your favorite dish to ensure it is safe for your diet.

living

Favorite Gluten-Free Holiday Recipes

I OFFER here several recipes to carry you through various holidays. Many foods associated with the holidays are thankfully already gluten-free—think cranberry relish, haroset, mashed potatoes, fudge—and others such as pumpkin pie only need to be slightly modified to make them gluten-free. Build on these recipes and you will find that the holidays are something to look forward to once again.

Favorite Fall Stuffing

LIKE BREAD pudding, good bread stuffing is often assumed to be unachievable in the gluten-free world. As we have discussed throughout this book, though, one of the essential keys to living a happy and successful gluten-free life is to try to make this new life feel nearly like the one you had before. That means that you should continue to eat out if that was your practice, you should entertain others and accept invitations for parties, and you should enjoy your old favorite foods made safe by being gluten-free. Therefore, if stuffing is as symbolic of Thanksgiving dinner to you as it is to me, you must find a way to have wonderful gluten-free bread stuffing at your table this year.

In my holiday gluten-free cooking classes, participants are starving for information on good gluten-free bread and stuffing. Most feel that they have been deprived of this Thanksgiving essential, having to substitute corn bread or even corn chips in other gluten-free stuffing attempts instead. There is absolutely nothing wrong with that approach nor with those results for something different; I just happen to crave the real bread stuffing I enjoyed in my former gluten-filled world, and so do most of them!

So in the spirit of Thanksgiving, I will share with you a gluten-free spin on traditional bread stuffings. My gluten-free "real bread" stuffing recipe also has the fun additions of flaxseed, fruit, and veggies for color, texture, and nutritional value. Feel free to add what you have on hand; make substitutions for or leave any of these extras out to suit your own tastes. You may bake your own gluten-free bread—or just dig out that presliced brick of store-bought gluten-free bread buried in your freezer (you know, the gift from well-meaning friends who thought they were doing you a favor?!). I like using those frozen commercial breads for stuffing because I covet my homemade gluten-free bread and hate to toast it when it is so good fresh! It seems a shame to take a delicious, fresh, moist loaf and cook all the yumminess out of it to make a stuffing, but great bread of course does make great stuffing! When I'm using the frozen kind, though, I feel as if I'm somehow recycling (rather than wasting food) and I enjoy the added benefit of getting extra space in my freezer!

Either way, I know you will enjoy this recipe and your Thanksgiving table will be blessed by the addition. (For more on gluten-free Thanksgiving ideas and gluten-free stuffing, listen to my radio interviews and articles updated on the Web site www.NearlyNormalCooking.com).

Makes enough for a full table of 6 to 8 to enjoy

6 cups gluten-free white bread cubes (do not use frozen bread sweetened with fruit juice)

1 tablespoon ground flaxseed

1/2 cup boiling water

1/2 cup butter or nondairy alternative

1 cup chopped carrots, turnips, and/or other root vegetables.

1/2 cup chopped celery

1/2 cup chopped onion

1/2 teaspoon grated nutmeg

1/4 teaspoon salt

1/4 teaspoon pepper

2 cups peeled, seeded, and chopped crisp apples, such as Gala, Fuji, or even Granny Smith

1/2 cup chopped pecans or walnuts

1/4 cup dried cranberries

1 cup gluten-free vegetable broth

1. Preheat the oven to 300°F.

2. Cut the bread slices into small cubes and spread in a single layer onto a cookie sheet. Bake for 10 to 15 minutes if using fresh bread or 5 to 10 minutes if using the previously frozen commercial variety, or until the cubes are dry but not burned.

3. In a small bowl, stir the flaxseed into the boiling water. Set aside to steep for 10 to 15 minutes.

4. In a large skillet, melt the butter, then add the vegetables and cook until tender. Add the nutmeg, salt, and pepper. Remove from the heat and set aside.

5. Place the dried bread cubes, chopped apples, nuts, berries, and flaxseed mixture in a large bowl and mix. Add the sautéed vegetables and stir well, then pour the entire mixture into a large baking dish with a lid. Pour most of the vegetable broth over the stuffing and stir, adding more broth as necessary to make a moist but not soupy stuffing. Cover and bake at 375°F for approximately 30 minutes, removing before it becomes too crispy.

Sweet Potato Soufflé

SWEET POTATOES are one of my perennial favorites and I use them in as many recipes as possible. The fall ushers in many excuses to bake with these root vegetables; sweet potato soufflé is the perfect side at your Thanksgiving table or an autumn potluck.

Serves 6

3 cups boiled, peeled, and mashed sweet potatoes (or use canned, drained, and mashed)

3/4 cup brown sugar

1/4 cup granulated sugar

1 egg, slightly beaten

1/2 cup milk (see text box on page 180 for dairy-free alternatives)

2 tablespoons melted butter or nondairy alternative

1 teaspoon gluten-free vanilla extract

1/2 teaspoon gluten-free almond flavoring

2 teaspoons ground cinnamon

3/4 cup grated sweetened coconut

Topping

1 cup brown sugar

4 tablespoons Nearly Normal All-Purpose Flour (page 48)

1/2 cup chopped pecans

1/2 cup grated coconut

4 tablespoons melted butter or nondairy alternative

1. Preheat the oven to 350°F. Butter or oil a 9 x 13-inch baking dish.

2. Mix all the ingredients except the topping in a bowl and pour into the prepared baking dish.

3. To prepare the topping, whisk together the dry ingredients in a bowl, then slowly stir in the melted butter. Spread the topping evenly over the soufflé and bake for 45 minutes, until cooked through.

Challah

I HAVE always loved this bread but never even attempted to make it in its wheat flour form. It looked too pretty to be easy, so I shied away from trying. Of course everything is a challenge with gluten-free baking at first, so eventually I figured, why not? My first concoction was such a success that I left it at that. Please do not be daunted as I was by this braided bread—this gluten-free recipe is easy to handle and comes out beautifully. You will be proud to serve this at the holidays.

Makes 2 braided loaves.

1/3 cup warm water

1 cup vanilla dairy or soy yogurt, at room temperature

1 teaspoon apple cider vinegar

5 large egg yolks, slightly beaten

1/3 cup canola oil

1/4 cup honey, agave nectar, or molasses

4 tablespoons granulated cane sugar

1 1/4 teaspoons salt

1/2 teaspoon baking soda

2 teaspoons gluten-free baking powder

4 cups Nearly Normal All-Purpose Flour (page 48)

2 1/2 teaspoons rapid rise gluten-free yeast (one 1/4-ounce envelope)

Cornstarch, for dusting

1 large egg, beaten, for brushing onto the loaves

Poppy seeds, sesame seeds, raisins, or other toppings or mix-ins

1. *If using bread machine:* Pour all the liquid ingredients into a bread machine set to the "Dough" setting. Next, add the sugar and then the remaining dry ingredients, saving the yeast. Make a well in the top of the dry ingredients and pour the yeast into the center. Close the lid and start the dough cycle. (If you choose to add raisins to the batter, add them during this cycle, after all the other ingredients have been mixed together.)

If using stand mixer: If you are not using a bread machine, add the ingredients together as listed and mix well using the dough hook attachment on your mixer.

Once the dough is mixed:

2. Preheat a warming drawer or your oven to 200°F, then turn off.

3. If using a bread machine, when the mixing portion of the cycle ends, you may remove the dough. Prepare a baking sheet by lining it with parchment paper.

4. Divide the dough in half and divide each half into three equal-size balls. Roll out each ball into a coil or long log on a clean, flat surface dusted with cornstarch. Pinch together one end of each coil, joining the three at the top, then braid them, finishing by pinching the other end together as well. You will then have one braided loaf. Gently transfer it to the parchment-lined baking sheet. Repeat for the second set of three balls.

5. Brush the beaten egg over each loaf well, coating the entire top surface. Sprinkle the seeds or any toppings at this point, then place the tray (covering the loaves with oiled waxed paper) in a warming drawer set to low heat, or into the preheated oven to rise for 20 to 30 minutes. (Don't expect the bread to rise much at this stage.)

6. Preheat the oven to 350°F. Place the uncovered tray in the oven and bake for 20 to 25 minutes. Remove to cool on a wire rack and cut after cooled.

Cherry Pie

MY GRANDMOTHER used to make the world's best berry pies. Fresh berries are crucial to making a really good pie, but I have found a few jarred varieties that are preserved in their own juices and make a mean pie. Please never even consider using canned pie filling . . . for anything. Aside from the possibility that a commercial filling contains gluten (check the labels), there is just no reason to settle for such mediocrity when a delicious berry pie is so easy to whip together. The hardest part about making a pie has always been the crust, not the filling. Follow this simple four-ingredient gluten-free pie crust recipe, refrigerate and moisten the dough, and your family will enjoy home-made, fresh, and heavenly cherry pie for their holiday festivities once again.

The key to all gluten-free dessert dough is to chill it before trying to work with it. Because of that, make sure to use enough water in the recipe so that the dough will not be dry and crumbly when you begin to roll it.

Grandma's Pie Crust Recipe (makes one 8- or 9-inch double pie crust)

2 cups Nearly Normal All-Purpose Flour (page 48)

1 teaspoon sea salt

2/3 cup Earth Balance Shortening (not Earth Balance Buttery Sticks)

5–6 tablespoons cold water

Cherry Pie Filling

4 cups cherries, pitted, stems removed

1/4 cup sugar

1/4 cup Nearly Normal All-Purpose Flour (page 48)

1. To prepare the crust: Mix the dry ingredients well, then cut in the shortening, using two knives or a pastry cutter. Add water to make the consistency you need to form two balls—ensure that the dough is not crumbly at this point, as refrigeration will dry it out further. Cover and refrigerate for at least 2 hours, until very cold.

2. Preheat the oven to 350°F. Remove one ball of cold dough and roll out the pastry onto a surface dusted with Nearly Normal All-Purpose Flour or cornstarch—I recommend using a flexible pastry mat or at minimum plastic wrap for that purpose. Turn the pie plate upside down on top of the rolled-out crust and flip the crust and plate over. Pat into shape.

3. Prepare the filling: In a bowl, combine all the cherry pie ingredients, mix well, and pour into the prepared crust.

4. For the top crust, roll out with the second ball of cold dough, covering it with plastic wrap so that it is sandwiched between the pastry mat and the plastic wrap. Turn the mat upside down and peel the crust off the mat (leaving it stuck to the plastic wrap on the other side). Lay the crust onto the pie filling and gently remove the plastic wrap from the top of the crust. Seal the two crusts together all around the rim with a small bit of cold water on your fingertips, pinching together to form scalloped edges. Place small pats of butter on top of the crust and sprinkle with cinnamon-sugar, if you desire.

2. Bake with the edges covered with foil or pie crust covers at 350°F for 20 to 30 minutes. Remove the foil and bake another 15 to 20 minutes, just until the top is lightly browned.

Crustless Coconut Pie

THIS PIE is an Easter family favorite, but once we make it, we remember how delicious it was, so I invariably end up making it several more times every spring! This pie requires no crust and it is delicious hot out of the oven, cold, or even at room temperature. I recommend doubling the recipe, because one pie is truly never enough. Another option is to bake in individual ramekins.

> 1½–2 cups of fresh or bagged sweetened flaked coconut
> 2 cups milk (see text box on page 180 for dairy-free alternatives)
> 4 eggs
> 1½ cups sugar
> ½ cup Nearly Normal All-Purpose Flour (page 48)
> 1 teaspoon gluten-free vanilla extract
> 8 tablespoons (1 stick) butter or nondairy alternative, melted

1. Preheat the oven to 350°F. Oil or butter a pie plate or ramekins.

2. Pour the coconut into a small bowl. Add the milk, stir, and set aside for at least 10 minutes to soak the coconut.

3. Beat the eggs and sugar in a large mixing bowl and add all the remaining ingredients slowly. Add the soaked coconut and pour into the prepared pie plate. This pie rises when cooking, then shrinks as it cools; therefore, be careful not to overfill the pie plate. I recommend leaving at least an inch clearance to allow for the pie to rise. Consequently, you may find that you have extra pie batter and will need to use an additional baking pan. This recipe also works well divided among several individual ramekins to serve guests.

4. Bake for 50 to 60 minutes (30 to 40 minutes if baking in ramekins), or until the edges are lightly browned and the middle is no longer jiggly.

Holiday Cut-Out Cookies

GROWING UP, nearly every "Hallmark holiday" in my house was an occasion to make cut-out cookies. Not just the big ones like Halloween, Christmas, and Valentine's Day, but even Groundhog Day sent me looking for the perfect food coloring and cookie cutter. As I searched for a gluten-free way of completing these holidays, I tried so many horrible rolled sugar cookie recipes that I nearly gave up. Finally I devised a gluten-free version of my old favorite that is easy to roll and cut, resilient, elastic, and yummy.

I often make this dough ahead of time and bring it out of the refrigerator (remember: with gluten-free dough, always refrigerate before working with it) for kids visiting on a playdate. For me, there's always a cookie holiday coming up, so this project is an easy and fun one for the kids that I can enjoy as well. One afternoon, another mother commented that she couldn't believe how many times we rolled the dough out to cut all the cookies (kids aren't the most efficient cookie cutters!), yet the dough never got crumbly or hard like her recipe (with gluten), so she wanted my gluten-free recipe. Prepare to double this recipe if you want to have enough to share.

$1/4$ cup Earth Balance Shortening
(not Earth Balance Buttery Sticks)

$2/3$ cup sugar

$1/4$ cup canola oil

2 egg yolks (look for pasteurized eggs so that if little
hands eat the dough, you can look the other way!)

2 teaspoons gluten-free vanilla extract

Food coloring (optional)

$13/4$ cups Nearly Normal All-Purpose Flour (page 48)

$1/2$ teaspoon salt

3 tablespoons water

Colored sugar (avoid using sprinkles, unless they are gluten-free) or
gluten-free frosting (optional)

1. Cream the shortening, sugar, and oil in a large bowl until fluffy. Add the egg yolks, vanilla extract, and food coloring, if using. Add the flour and salt, alternating with as much water as necessary to achieve the desired consistency:

a moist but not wet cookie dough. Refrigerate for at least 2 to 3 hours, if possible. It is important that the dough be cold when you work with it, so freeze it if you are in a big rush and need to make the cookies right away.

2. Preheat the oven to 350°F. Line a baking sheet with parchment paper.

3. Lightly flour the rolling surface and rolling pin with Nearly Normal All-Purpose Flour or cornstarch, and dust the cookie cutters, too, before using to cut shapes. Roll the dough to approximately 1/8-inch thickness.

4. Place the cut-out cookies onto the prepared baking sheet and decorate with colored sugar, if desired. Bake for 8 to 10 minutes, until the cookies begin to lightly brown at the edges. Transfer to a rack to cool. When baked and cooled, use gluten-free frosting to decorate, if desired.

IN A SENTENCE

> *Holidays are for celebrating, reflecting, and honoring—whatever the occasion, gluten-free participants needn't miss a moment of these special times if we simply revise tried-and-true recipes, host the get-togethers, and invite others to duplicate our gluten-free recipes for future occasions.*

MONTH 10

Advanced Gluten-Free Baking

BY NOW, you've become accustomed to following gluten-free recipes and you have a feel for how to handle gluten-free dough and batter. Converting regular wheat flour recipes to gluten-free recipes is the next step in your gluten-free transition.

As you now know, no single gluten-free flour can successfully replace wheat flour by itself. Therefore, a mixture of alternative flours is necessary to mimic the performance of traditional wheat flours. In recipes that are not gluten-free, your all-purpose mix will be used as if it were a wheat flour and the amounts will be the same. Some adjustments might have to be made to effect a seamless transition to gluten-free for wheat flour recipes, but the flour amount should remain the same, making you free to convert all of your old favorite recipes to gluten-free.

Here, I have outlined in more detail some of the many alternative flours available to you, now that you are cooking gluten-free. You should experiment with these to see if you prefer one mixture for bread and another for cookies, for example, and to find ones that suit your tastes. As I mentioned, it is totally possible to use the same recipe as an "all-purpose" mixture if it works for you in all of your baking (see page 48 for my personal all-purpose recipe); it is just nice to know that if you ever get ambitious, have extra time, are curious about other grains, develop other dietary requirements, or just plain want a change, you have options!

Alternative Gluten-Free Flours

Almond Flour: Made from finely ground almonds, this rich-tasting nut flour is very high in protein and provides a wonderfully smooth taste to breads, cakes, and cookies. Due to the high protein and fat content of almond flour, it should be refrigerated or frozen. Do not buy or make more than you can reasonably use, as this flour is very expensive.

Amaranth Flour: A high-protein, starchy flour with a strong, nutty taste, this tiny seed looks like couscous in its natural form. Amaranth was a key crop to the ancient Aztec society and offers a rich supply of calcium and iron. Use in combination with other gluten-free flours in such foods as pancakes, quick breads, or muffins, but be cautious about using it in large proportions, as it can cause baked goods to brown more quickly, leaving the dough on the inside undercooked. Store in the refrigerator.

Arrowroot Powder: Used like cornstarch or cream of tartar, this starch thickens sauces and provides stability. This starch is extracted from the roots of various plants most often native to Central America. Arrowroot starch is very similar to tapioca starch and is also easily digested. It is very soft and tender and needs to be combined with other flours when baking, for body.

Brown Rice Flour: Higher nutritional content than its white rice flour counterpart, it also is typically grittier. It is available in health food stores and larger supermarkets that carry alternative grains. Store it in the refrigerator.

Buckwheat Flour: Not related to wheat, buckwheat is actually related to rhubarb. Buckwheat groats are the kernel inside the inedible outer hull. Roasted buckwheat groats are called "kasha." Buckwheat noodles ("soba" noodles) are a nice alternative to spaghetti or rice noodles. Buckwheat in any of its forms offers high protein, stability, and a sweet, nutty flavor that accents many pancakes and muffins.

Chickpea Flour: Chickpeas (garbanzo beans) are high in protein and absorb liquid when cooked. Chickpea flour (also known as "gram" flour, not to be confused with "graham") has a distinctive bean taste if used in large proportions but offers good bread structure as well.

Coconut Flour: A rich-tasting flour with extra fiber and a unique sweet taste. A nice alternative to bean flours when looking for higher-fiber flours in desserts, although it can be difficult to find. Coconut readily absorbs moisture, so you may need to adjust the proportions of the liquids or flours you mix it with. Should be stored in the refrigerator or freezer.

Corn Flour: Corn flour is simply the finest grade of cornmeal (not the same as cornstarch). You can make your own corn flour by grinding corn meal in a blender or food processor. Corn flour and cornmeal offer a crunchy texture and a dense, firm structure to breads and breakfast foods like pancakes; both are inexpensive and easily available in grocery stores and Latin American specialty grocers. Corn flour and corn meal also offer fiber and fat to add nutritional value to your baked goods.

Cornstarch: Ubiquitous in mainstream grocery stores, this very fine, light starch has no distinctive flavors, fat, or fiber but provides great thickening properties.

Flaxseed Meal: The ancient crop of flax can be traced back to ancient Egypt. Ground flaxseeds are notably high in fiber, minerals, and antioxidants and they yield a nutty flavor and texture to baked goods. Flaxseeds steeped in boiling water can even be used in place of eggs to retain structure in breads. The seeds and meal should be refrigerated or frozen.

Garfava Flour: A unique high-protein combination of garbanzo bean (chickpea) and fava flour that offers a milder bean taste than garbanzo bean flour on its own. (Some people are highly allergic to fava beans and need to avoid this combination.) The flour should be stored in the refrigerator or freezer.

Millet Flour: This bland flour becomes rancid quickly, so grind your own or freeze your stock of flour to preserve it. Millet has long been a staple in Africa and millet flakes can be used to make porridge. It is high in iron.

Oat Flour: Certified gluten-free oats and oat flour are now available and offer fiber, protein, and texture often lacking in other gluten-free flours. Store oat flakes or flour in the refrigerator, freezer, or an airtight container. A small percentage of celiacs may not tolerate oats, even if they are certified gluten-free. Check with your own physician before introducing oats into your gluten-free diet.

Oat Bran: This product is the outer casing of the oat grain, which contains valuable soluble fiber. When certified gluten-free, it can be a tasty addition to quick breads and cookies or a useful component to coating fish or chicken.

Other Nut Flours: Hazelnut, chestnut, and other nut flours add rich flavor and smooth texture to gluten-free recipes. Replace up to one-quarter of the flour in any recipe with nut flours alone, but balance with an all-purpose gluten-free flour containing xanthan or guar gum for stability. You may grind your own nut flours using a spice grinder. Store any unused nut flours in the refrigerator or freezer, due to the high oil content of most nut flours except for chestnut.

Potato Flour: A heavy, mild flour that absorbs moisture in recipes, providing stability. However, this cannot be used in high proportion, due to its moisture-robbing qualities. Has been dubbed by one food testing company as "the safest food in Britain," as it is extremely well tolerated by most people.[1]

Potato Starch: Sometimes referred to as "potato starch flour," the starch of the potato is a wonderful thickening agent that offers a smooth, flavor-free base to any all-purpose mix. When used in combination with other gluten-free flours, it may add volume and softness to gluten-free breads.

Quinoa Flour: Recently enjoying a resurgence in popularity, quinoa is an ancient, grainlike seed. It is remarkably high in protein and amino acids and lends a nutty taste to foods. Try cooking it instead of rice as a side dish.

Sorghum Flour: A nice all-purpose grain common in African and Indian baking. It is a good go-to grain when making substitutions in all-purpose mixes due to other grain sensitivities. Sorghum is also a good source of insoluble fiber.

Soy Flour: A high-protein flour made from dried and ground soybeans. This heavy ingredient adds bulk to all-purpose mixes but is difficult for some people to digest. Used in large proportion, it can leave a detectable aftertaste and causes foods to brown more quickly than with other flours. Store it in the refrigerator or freezer.

Tapioca Starch or Flour: This smooth flour is extracted from a root known as "cassava," "manioc," or "yucca"; it is smooth and flavorless but adds chewy texture to baked goods and is a good thickener. Like arrowroot, it is very delicate and should be combined with other flours for body, when baking.

---

1. "Potato Is Best Tolerated Food, Says Tester," Food Navigator.com: Breaking News on Food & Beverage Development–Europe, http://www.foodnavigator.com/news/printNewsBis.asp?id=83070.

Teff Flour: Highly nutritious and high fiber, teff provides a sweet nutty flavor.

White Rice Flour: Long the standby flour for gluten-free baking, white rice flour offers bulk without flavor or much nutritional value. It is available in very finely ground form, particularly in Latin American or Asian markets.

Gluten-free flours all tend to absorb more moisture than do their wheat flour counterparts, so it is important to bear in mind that additional moisture will be needed in most recipes to avoid drying them out. By the same token, you do not want to store your gluten-free flours in a moist environment. If your canisters are sealed well, you should be able to leave most of these flours in your cupboard or pantry, but higher-fat flours from such things as wild rice, dried beans, nuts, and seeds should be refrigerated or frozen if you plan on keeping them for a longer period of time.

Binding Agents

In addition, a binding agent such as xanthan gum or guar gum is required to replace the elasticity and structure of gluten. I have found that xanthan gum works nicely in most all recipes, but guar gum is slightly better in cakes. In my cooking classes, I have met some celiacs with sensitivities to guar gum, though, so I almost exclusively use xanthan gum when preparing samples or consulting with newly diagnosed celiacs. Bear in mind as well that guar gum has much higher fiber than does xanthan, so if you choose to use guar, expect that some laxative effects may occur with larger measurements. Other alternative binders offering success in gluten-free baking include mung bean (a.k.a. green bean) flour and pregelled potato flour (but this can be difficult to find). Both of these flours are bulkier additions than the gums, requiring approximately ⅛ cup to each cup of gluten-free flour; adjust the wet ingredients in your recipes accordingly.

Another interesting product recently released into the gluten-free marketplace is Expandex®, a modified tapioca starch with binding and leavening abilities. The manufacturer recommends using this starch to reduce or even eliminate the use of gums in your gluten-free baking.[2] I now use Expandex in my own all-purpose mix, as I have found that with Expandex, I can reduce the amount of xanthan gum; the mixture also provides the added benefit of

---

2. http://www.expandexglutenfree.com/.

extending the shelf stability of my baked foods. I often bake bread made with Expandex and store it out of the refrigerator for many days at a time, with no spoiling or drying effects. Products such as Expandex are welcome additions to your gluten-free baking shelf, either by themselves or found as ingredients in premixed gluten-free items.

Leavening Agents

Successful gluten-free baking usually requires additional leavening agents as well. Initial experiments should incorporate extra baking powder, baking soda, or yeast, depending on the recipe. Furthermore, egg whites, gelatin, flaxseed meal, or dry milk powder added to your recipes will help to stabilize the food when it rises and will reduce the kind of cave-ins often experienced with breads, cakes, and muffins. You will notice in the recipes I have provided for you in this book that I often use these tips to create my own recipes. Extrapolate from my measurements to devise gluten-free proportions for your own new recipes.

The Starch-to-Flour Ratio

If you decide to create your own flour mix recipe, recognize that when selecting from the many alternative gluten-free flours available, some are lighteners (usually starches), and others add bulk instead; you should be looking to create a mixture that does both. Your ultimate gluten-free mixture should have an approximate starch-to-flour ratio of between 3:2 and 5:4, and you should add approximately ¾ to 1 teaspoon of xanthan or guar gum to each cup of flour mix. If you are indeed making different mixes for each type of baked product you create (you have more time and energy than I!), you should be using slightly less gum for cookies and more for breads, with cakes falling somewhere in the middle.

Substituting Your All-Purpose Flour
Mix in a Gluten-Free Recipe

So, once you have an all-purpose mix that you are comfortable using in most recipes, understand that many gluten-free recipes you find in cookbooks will break out into individual flours and gums the ingredients required for that particular recipe. Rather than follow the recipe's call for 1 cup of this flour and ½ cup of that starch and 1 teaspoon of xanthan gum, simply add the amounts of each flour in the list to derive a total amount of flours and starches and gums for the recipe—in this example, 1½ cups + 1 teaspoon. Now use that same total amount of your all-purpose gluten-free mix instead.

The transition only gets tricky when the gluten-free recipe you are using either calls for a lot of starches or a lot of bulkier flours, and thus falls out of the starch-to-flour ratio range you have in your mixture. For these recipes, you may find that your all-purpose mix is not the appropriate balance. I have supplied an illustration in the text box to explain this problem; fortunately, this difficulty arises only rarely.

Balancing Flour and Starch

Problem: A gluten-free recipe you would like to try calls for 2 cups of starch and 1 cup of brown rice flour. Your all-purpose gluten-free flour mix contains 1 cup of starch, 1 cup of quinoa flour, and 1 cup of amaranth flour. The recipe calls for a 2:1 starch-to-flour ratio, whereas your mix has a 1:2 starch-to-flour ratio.

Solution: This recipe requires a lighter mix than you are using, so you can either simply follow the recipe as it is written, or use 1½ cups of starch and 1½ cups of your flour mix to equal the same starch-to-flour ratio.

Note: Your only other real concern at this point would be adding enough gum to equal the amount called for in the recipe, since adding simple starch (as opposed to your all-purpose mix) will not contain any binding agents. In a cookie recipe, this deficiency would likely not be noticeable; however, in a loaf of bread, the difference could make or break the recipe.

IN A SENTENCE

Many gluten-free grains are available and, if you have any additional dietary concerns or the desire to simply try some new flavors, you should feel free to expand your gluten-free grain horizons.

living

Baking and Breaking Gluten-Free Bread

THERE ARE a couple of mistaken "truths" about gluten-free breads, which have for the most part been held as self-evident and universal. The first is that all gluten-free bread is dry, dense, and crumbly. This is absolutely not true, although most commercially available frozen loaves do fit this description. In this chapter, I provide recipes for bread, rolls, biscuits, and other yeast and quick breads that will satisfy the most discriminating bread eaters in your family and disprove the bad reputation gluten-free bread has earned.

The second is that gluten-free bread falls or caves in when it is removed from the oven to cool. Again, not all recipes yield these unsatisfactory results. Additions such as eggs, milk powder, gelatin, and even flaxseed meal can help your breads resist cave-ins. Purchasing pans that are deep enough to support the sides of your loaves during baking and cooling can also help. The recipes I give you in this chapter will help you produce breads that not only taste delicious but offer aesthetic appeal as well. As a general gluten-free rule of thumb, though, because of fluctuating moisture levels in gluten-free flours, you may find that occasionally your breads will sink. If your yeast breads cave in, decrease the liquid by 3 tablespoons or try this flaxseed trick: Dissolve 2 tablespoons of flaxseed meal in ¼ cup of boiling water. Steep for 10 minutes, then add into your recipe. Decrease the liquids in your existing recipe proportionately.

Finally, even many expert bread bakers are afraid of gluten-free bread recipes. I remember a particular celiac disease benefit where the professional caterer refused to bake gluten-free bread for the large and prestigious crowd. I offered my bread sticks recipe, using my flour mixture, to another caterer who agreed to try it first, before agreeing to prepare the bread sticks for the event. When the samples had been produced and tasted, the caterer gladly signed on to prepare the bread sticks at the event because they were so delicious, moist, and savory. Compliments abounded that evening, and hopefully the lesson learned by everyone (including the caterer) was that making delicious gluten-free breads with mass appeal is not only possible, it is relatively easy!

Experiment with these wonderful yeast and quick bread recipes for yourself, and add nearly normal breads back to your family's menu.

Nearly Normal Southern Biscuits

ONE OF the things I have missed most in my gluten-free life is biscuits—buttery, light, and fluffy biscuits like I remember from my childhood in the South and from favorite drive-throughs like Bojangles' and Biscuitville. As with every other gluten-free challenge, I determined to tackle this one successfully, and I think you'll appreciate the results.

Makes 9 biscuits

2 cups Nearly Normal All-Purpose
Flour (page 48)

2 teaspoons gluten-free baking
powder

$1/2$ teaspoon baking soda

1 teaspoon coarse sea salt, or
$1/2$ teaspoon fine sea salt plus
$1/2$ teaspoon coarse sea salt

4 tablespoons butter, plus additional
butter to spread on the tops
before baking

$1/4$ cup dry buttermilk powder, or
$1/4$ dry milk powder plus
$1/2$ teaspoon apple cider vinegar
added to the half-and-half, below

$1/2$ cup half-and-half

$1/2$ cup regular or light sour cream

Potato starch or cornstarch,
for dusting

1. Preheat the oven to 350°F if convection (preferred) or 375°F if non-convection. Line a baking sheet with parchment paper.

2. Whisk together the dry ingredients in a large bowl. Cut the butter into the dry ingredients with a pastry cutter or two knives, until you achieve the consistency of coarse meal. Add the half-and-half and sour cream, and stir with a fork to thoroughly combine.

3. Pat the dough onto a lightly floured (with potato starch or cornstarch) counter or pastry mat, forming a 6- to 7-inch disk approximately 1 inch thick. Dip a biscuit cutter into your potato starch or cornstarch and cut out nine biscuits (cut straight down, do not twist the cutter).

4. Transfer to the prepared baking sheet and prick the tops with a fork a few times. Lay a small, thin pat of butter on the top of each biscuit before baking.

5. Bake for approximately 14 minutes, or until the tops are lightly browned and they are firm but not hard. It is important not to overbake them.

Nutty White Bread (without the nuts!)

THIS RECIPE, which may be made without eggs and/or dairy, may be prepared using a mixer and oven or in a bread machine. This loaf is light and airy, yet substantial enough to use as sandwich bread. It also boasts the addition of flaxseed meal and flaxseeds, which contribute a large amount of dietary fiber and other beneficial nutritional properties, such as high omega–3 fatty acids. The simple addition of two tablespoons of flaxseed meal to this bread adds four grams of dietary fiber and three grams of protein. As an alternative, you can simply use two eggs in place of the flaxseed mixture, and you will not be proofing the yeast.

2 tablespoons ground flaxseed or flaxseed meal

$1/2$ cup very hot water

1 tablespoon rapid-rise or bread machine yeast

1 tablespoon granulated cane sugar

$31/4$ cups Nearly Normal All-Purpose Flour (page 48)

$1/2$ teaspoon baking soda

2 teaspoons gluten-free baking powder

Pinch of salt

1 tablespoon whole flaxseeds, sunflower seeds, or coarsly ground nuts like pecans

$1/4$ cup Earth Balance Shortening, cut into small pieces, or canola oil if using a breadmaker

1 teaspoon apple cider vinegar

2 tablespoons honey

1 cup vanilla dairy or soy yogurt

Cooking oil spray

Toppings of choice (coarse sea salt, sesame seeds, flaxseeds, etc.)

To prepare in a conventional oven:

1. In a small bowl, combine the flaxseed meal and hot water and stir. Let sit for 5 minutes. Add the yeast and sugar to this mixture and stir. Set aside for 5 more minutes.

2. Sift the remaining dry ingredients together (except do not add the yeast yet) in a large bowl. Add the pieces of shortening and mix, using a pastry cutter or the dough paddle on your mixer. Add the cider vinegar, honey, and yogurt, mixing well. Finally, mix in the yeast mixture and stir well, using the dough paddle.

3. Oil a bread pan (use a dark metal pan if you like a darker crust on your bread; lighter, shiny metal or glass if you like a light crust). Scoop the dough into the pan. Smooth the top, then cover with a sheet of waxed paper sprayed with cooking oil. Sit the covered dough for 30 minutes in a warm place, such as an oven warming drawer or even in your oven with the light on. Preheat a convection oven (preferred) to 275°F or a nonconvection oven to 300°F.

4. Add your desired toppings and place the raised dough in the preheated oven. Bake for approximately 30 minutes, or until the crust is browning nicely and a cake tester or skewer inserted into the center of the loaf comes out clean. Remove to a cooling rack and rotate gently from side to side every 5 minutes or so, to prevent excessive sinking in the middle of the loaf. When cooled for 15 minutes or more, remove from the loaf pan to finish cooling before slicing.

When using a bread machine: Always be sure to add all liquid ingredients to the pan first, followed by the dry ingredients. I recommend sifting all dry ingredients together in a bowl first, then pouring it into the bread machine pan. Reserve the yeast for last in bread machines, making a small well in the top of the dry ingredients in the pan and pouring the yeast into that well. Select either the gluten-free bread setting on your machine, or the quickest bake setting, such as for a light crust 1½-pound loaf. Remove the pan from the machine as soon as it is finished baking.

Bread Sticks

THIS IS one of my most flexible go-to recipes. You can use these same ingredients for dinner rolls, soft pretzels, cinnamon buns, or breadsticks. Go crazy and get creative with shapes and toppings.

1 teaspoon apple cider vinegar

1/4 cup Earth Balance Shortening

3 tablespoons honey

2 eggs

1 cup vanilla dairy or soy yogurt

2 cups Nearly Normal All-Purpose Flour (page 48)

1/2 teaspoon baking soda

2 teaspoons gluten-free baking powder

Pinch of salt

1 tablespoon rapid-rise yeast

Potato starch or cornstarch, for dusting

Topping(s) of choice

1. Preheat the oven to 350°F. Line a baking sheet with parchment paper.

2. Combine the wet ingredients in a large bowl and gradually add the dry ingredients, saving the yeast for last and mixing with a dough hook until the lumps are removed from the dough.

3. Dust the counter with potato starch or cornstarch and some of your toppings. Dust your hands with the starch as well. Grab chunks of the wet dough, rolling it in the starch and topping(s) into the shape you desire. Lay the sticks, pretzels, or other shaped dough onto the prepared baking sheet. Sprinkle with the remaining topping(s) and bake for 10 to 12 minutes, until the tops are lightly browned and the dough has risen.

Southern Corn Bread

EACH WEEK I post at least one new recipe in my blog at www.NearlyNormal Cooking.com. On more than one occasion, I have suggested serving corn bread with a particular soup, jambalaya, or other meal offering and provide my tried and true "Southern Corn Bread" recipe. This posting invariably elicits a running commentary from readers who contend either that this is the absolute best corn bread that they have ever tasted, or that it is not truly "Southern" because there is too much sugar. Whatever your particular position on the subject, I have never heard a complaint about the taste.

So, here is my controversial, yet always crowd-pleasing, corn bread recipe. If you feel very strongly about it, simply cut back on the recommended amount of sugar.

> 1 tablespoon oil or butter, if prepping a cast-iron skillet
> 3/4 cup Nearly Normal All-Purpose Flour (page 48)
> 1 teaspoon salt
> 1/2 teaspoon baking soda
> 1 tablespoon baking powder
> 3/4 cup cornmeal
> 3/4 cup sugar
> 1 cup milk or soy milk
> 1 egg or egg-free alternative
> 1/4 cup vanilla dairy or soy yogurt
> 1/4 teaspoon apple cider vinegar

1. Preheat the oven to 375°F. Grease an 8-inch square baking pan (or, if using a cast-iron skillet, put 1 tablespoon of oil or butter in the skillet and place in the oven to preheat).

2. To mix the ingredients, wisk together all the dry ingredients in a bowl and set aside. Next, mix all liquid ingredients in a large bowl, using a mixer or a whisk, then add the dry ingredients slowly, mixing until the bigger lumps are removed. The batter should be thin but not watery.

3. Pour into your prepared pan (if not using a cast-iron skillet) and place in the oven, or remove the skillet from the oven using baking mitts, and pour

the batter into the pan, returning it to the oven to bake for approximately 30 minutes. The top and edges will be nicely but lightly browned, and a cake tester inserted into the center of the pan will be clean. Do not overbake! Serve from the skillet or pan by cutting into pie wedges.

IN A SENTENCE

> *Delicious and appealing gluten-free breads are indeed possible and are worth the effort, as you can always produce better breads fresh than what you can obtain frozen at your grocer.*

MONTH **11**

learning

"I Need a Vacation!"

ALL THIS baking, entertaining, and partying will take its toll if you let it, and everyone deserves a vacation every now and again. Do not let fears of gluten exposure shackle you to your home and your tried-and-true restaurants. Celiac disease just may be the ticket to a whole new world of travel for you.

Gluten-Free Travel Clubs

A diagnosis of celiac disease led a couple in Maryland to form a gluten-free travel club in 1995, through which thousands of celiacs have found they can safely travel the world. Bob and Ruth's Gluten-Free Dining and Travel Club (www.bobandruths.com) began after Bob Levy was diagnosed with celiac disease in the mid-1990s. He had actually been diagnosed as an infant and became a "Banana Baby" like Barbara Hudson (see Day 5). He was told that he was "cured" as a child, on the banana diet, and went on to live a seemingly healthy and normal life until becoming sick with diagnosed celiac disease in his fifties.

After gaining confidence with the gluten-free diet, Bob and his wife, Ruth, began to travel the world; the dining and travel club evolved out of his passionate pursuit of safe gluten-free travel.

Now they take five to seven trips all over the world every year, in addition to two- or three-night mini-getaways in the United States. Gluten-free travelers and their companions of all ages and nationalities have joined them on these well-planned adventures to everywhere from African safaris to Club Med and European river cruises. Lavish gluten-free meals are planned with executive chefs well in advance, and the chefs and waitstaff are introduced to the group before every meal, to further ensure food safety. Apparently, these trips are so much fun that up to half of the travelers return to enjoy more vacations.

This type of adventure is an opportunity to meet others who have celiac in common—instant friendships are formed and fond memories are made because of, not in spite of, celiac disease. If you are hesitant to travel or fearful to venture out of English-speaking regions, consider a planned trip such as this to jump-start you to your own gluten-free travels. Children also benefit from being with others who have celiac disease in common. Many camps have sprung up recently, offering summertime fun for celiac children in a range of age groups. The Gluten Intolerance Group is a good resource for lists of this type of camp offered all over the country. For more information or to register online, go to www.gluten.net/events.htm.

Agencies and Tours

Other preplanned travel options geared toward celiacs include cruise lines, dude ranches, and bed-and-breakfasts. Several travel agencies actually specialize in helping gluten-free travelers find suitable accommodations. Gluten-Free Travel (www.glutenfreetravel.com.au) offers a portal into cruise lines, tours, planned trips, or simple travel agency services around the world that cater to gluten-free travelers. Other sites, such as http://glutenfreeonthego.com/default.asp, also offer some help in locating cruise lines, places to stay, and restaurants that serve gluten-free food, internationally.

Do not feel as if you must travel with others, or with other celiacs, to travel safely; if group travel is not for you, apply your acquired knowledge of gluten-free living to any trip you plan. Try your own Internet searches with your destination in mind (for example, before traveling to Russia, visit www.celiac.spb.ru/eng.htm). Review the content available on user-friendly free search engines, such as www.celiachandbook.com/, where you can locate restaurants around the world that serve gluten-free food. For European travel planning, be sure to visit the Web site of the Association of European Coeliac

Societies (AOECS), at www.aoecs.org/. This site maintains free listings of e-mail addresses and Web sites for all its European Celiac Society members; each country's own site contains additional information unique to travel in that particular country.

Carry Cook Cards and Keep Snacks on Hand

Take advantage of the free printable cook cards offered by many listed country sites in their native languages, as well as listings of shops and restaurants that serve gluten-free visitors. No matter where you travel, you should always carry this type of cook card. Review or print the one shown on page 120 of this book for a free starter card. For additional translations of this type of card, visit www.celiactravel.com/restaurant-cards.html, which provides thirty-eight translated cards for a voluntary donation; or www.glutenfreepassport.com/traveling/translations.html, which also offers a "Multi-Lingual Phrase Passport" for a fee, ordered directly from their Web site. Particularly when visiting other countries, having confidence in communicating with restaurant staff is key to enjoying your meals and your travel.

However, as my mother always says, pack extras "just in case," so whether I am traveling stateside or abroad, I always pack a gallon-size resealable plastic bag full of gluten-free snack bars such as Bora Bora bars (www.wellements .com/borabars.asp) or Larabars (www.larabar.com/secure/index_.php), as well as nuts and trail mix in individual bags. Having snacks on hand for any kind of travel ensures that you can at least nosh your way safely through the day on any trip.

◇ ◇ ◇

Traveling Just Got Easier! Bonnie Sysko's Story

I find that breakfast is the most difficult meal during travel, since I enjoy cereal and have never found gluten-free cereals in restaurants. I often fill plastic bags with cereal, packing them along with gluten-free snacks for each day of travel. I always keep food handy in my pocketbook and, when flying to any destination, I bring a snack for the time spent at the airport and on the plane, because finding gluten-free foods in that situation can be a challenge. When flying to visit family and friends and staying at their homes, I request that they pick up some gluten-free foods for me before my arrival.

When traveling by car, I am able to take more gluten-free foods along, thus freeing up time to visit that would otherwise be used to shop for foods. On occasion I have prepared and frozen meals, placing them in a cooler aimed for my destination. My meal can then be warmed, taking little or no effort by the hostess, yet providing me a safe meal while others are eating what I cannot. By doing some research and preparation before my trip, I can relax during the time I am gone, because I know I will not be searching for safe choices. I can still totally enjoy what I am doing, and with whom I am doing it. I do not dwell on what I cannot eat each day. I focus on everything else I can do.

◇ ◇ ◇

Food Restrictions Will Not Hold Me Back! Chrissy Andrews's Story

Recently, I decided to study abroad in Dublin, Ireland. At first I procrastinated in applying for the program, and I realized it was due to anxiety about eating safely in another country for several months. However, I researched my options online and, to my delight, I discovered that there is a more extensive awareness of the disease in Ireland than in the United States. Gluten-free options are readily available in many of the restaurants and marked clearly on menus. It's amazing the amount of information you can gain from the Internet. Although I will never drink a Guinness in an Irish pub, hard cider (gluten-free, of course!) is available on tap in almost every pub in Ireland! I realize that I will have to put a little extra effort into figuring out my meals in Ireland than will the typical student, and traveling to other countries (especially Italy—so much pizza and pasta!) will present additional problems, but I am confident that I will be able to successfully survive abroad and I will not let my food restrictions hold me back from living my life.

◇ ◇ ◇

IN A SENTENCE

> *Take the opportunity to explore the world and spread the word while you are traveling to pave the way for others; whatever you do, do not let fears of contamination hold you back from living life to its fullest at home or abroad.*

living

My Best Travel Tips:
Michele Wallick's Story

YOU MAY never meet anyone who travels more than Michele Wallick—celiac or otherwise. Yet Michele's zest for living, wherever she happens to be, should inspire us all as celiacs and demonstrate that we are only limited by the size and destinations of our dreams. Michele simply refuses to be constrained by celiac disease, and so should you!

◇ ◇ ◇

Michele Wallick's Story

My name is Michele Wallick and I was diagnosed with celiac disease in December 2006. As a mechanical engineer, former vice president in a major consulting firm, and entrepreneur, I have always been consumed by traveling around the world. My husband and I now travel to scuba dive, sail, ski, hike, and ride our tandem bicycle. We are currently preparing for two months of travel through various parts of Africa and will then sail across the Atlantic to Brazil. Celiac disease has not slowed me down or restricted my travel. It has made me into a travel planner, has caused me to ask lots of questions, and has driven me to push the international boundaries of gluten-free foods. Everywhere I go now is a new gluten-free adventure where I educate others on celiac disease and gluten-free, and I steel my resolve to never give up on my passion for living life to its fullest.

If I wasn't already, I have learned since my diagnosis to become completely self-reliant. For gluten-free travel purposes, this can mean many different things. On one end of the spectrum, self-reliance can be defined as carrying all your food with you everywhere you go. On the other end of the spectrum, self-reliance can be defined as finding access to grocery stores and knowing how to work with restaurant staff to ensure that they feed you safely.

Mastering gluten-free travel to me is accepting that I've now become a kind of "inspector gadget" with all my various gluten-free food containers. Whether it is "routine" travel for work, vacation, meeting friends for dinner, or holiday feasts, every day is a new opportunity for a gluten-free adventure. Here are some of the solutions I have developed; I hope they encourage you to travel freely as well.

Tip #1—All Containers Are Not Created Equal

Thermos. The Thermos company (www.thermos.com) makes a microwavable food jar that keeps food hot for four hours and keeps food cold for six. As a ski instructor, I'm always looking for new ideas of what to eat for lunch. Since ski resorts do not often sell many gluten-free options, I pack my lunch every day in my backpack. Even though this thermos is bulky, it's perfect for my gluten-free beef stew, soups, or chowders. I microwave my food right inside the container in the morning, and then I have a warm lunch on a cold winter day.

Insulated bags. Insulated soft-sided bags or the thermo-snap bags from grocery stores work really well for traveling. Because of airline regulations, you are not able to have a frozen gel pack in your carry-on luggage. However, a bag of frozen vegetables or even frozen gluten-free lunch meats work really well to keep your food cold, and these bags will pass inspection at the airport. Even after all my many flights, no one has ever confiscated my frozen peas! This solution also yields you extra food to eat once the bag has defrosted, so be sure to choose your own favorite bag of frozen food.

Plastic containers. Using resealable bags versus plastic containers should be determined by the consistency and texture of your food. For example, nuts can easily travel in a resealable bag. However, rice crackers usually need something sturdy, such as a plastic container. There are many brands of containers in a variety of sizes. I'll usually have large plastic containers in my suitcase and the smaller containers in my bag or backpack. My favorite airtight brand is Lock&Lock (www.locknlock.com.au/history.htm). You can find many sizes at Target, Wal-Mart, and supermarkets. The only thing you need to watch when you're washing the container is safely getting the O-ring out of the lid without scoring the rubber.

Tip #2—Research Airline Regulations and Services

It's important to understand airport regulations and to research what gluten-free food is offered by your airline. Particularly after 9/11, these regulations now seem to change rather frequently, so you need to double-check with your carrier before you leave. I have also heard many stories about the airlines mixing up the gluten-free meals with other special meals that may not be gluten-free. Make sure that you introduce yourself to the flight attendants and stress the importance of your gluten-free meal. Never trust that the regular airline meal will be gluten-free.

Below is a list of some major U.S. airlines and their gluten-free status as of March 2008. As with food labels, always recheck with your airline before your flight, since the foods they offer are likely to change.

AirTran Airways (800) AIR-TRAN—Non-gluten-free pretzels are the only snack served on all their flights. No full meals are served.

American Airlines (800) 433-7300—Gluten-free meals are offered with advance notice. Different snack options vary from flight to flight.

Continental Airlines (800) 932-2732—Gluten-free is considered a "special" meal request. There are only selected flights that offer "special" meal requests. Therefore, there are certain flights where only non-gluten-free meals are offered.

Delta Airlines (800) 221-1212—Delta recommends that you talk to a representative over the phone to order your gluten-free meal. Different snack options vary from flight to flight.

JetBlue Airlines (800) 538-2583—JetBlue offers a variety of snacks, but only the cashews are gluten-free. No full meals are served.

Northwest Airlines (701) 420-6282—Snacks/meals are listed on their Web site—and none are gluten-free. Please call for more information.

Southwest Airlines (800) I-FLY-SWA—Various snacks are offered, but peanuts are your only gluten-free option. However, if someone on your flight has a peanut allergy, no peanuts will be served to anyone and you would need to bring your own snack.

US Airways (800) 428-4322—There is no guarantee of gluten-free snacks. However, you may order a gluten-free meal in advance for international flights.

United Airlines (800) UNITED-1—Gluten pretzels are the only snack on domestic flights in coach. However, business or first-class passengers often have nuts as an option that is not available for coach passengers. Gluten-free meals can be ordered for international flights in advance.

Tip #3—Develop an Airport Strategy

You should first understand the shelf-stable and nonperishable food/snack options that are appropriate for carrying on a plane. Also keep in mind that your plane may be delayed or you may miss a connecting flight. I always have backup food just in case I need to eat safely. Below are some ideas for possible airport travel food.

GF Pretzels
GF Crackers
GF Cheese (depending on temperature and conditions)
GF Yogurt (depending on temperature and conditions)
Vegetables (carrots, celery, cherry tomatoes, etc.)
Fruit (apple, banana, orange, etc.)
Peanut Butter/Jelly (travel size)
GF Rice Noodle Dishes
GF Lunch Meat
GF Beef Jerky
GF Olives
GF Snack Bars
Nuts
GF Cereal in a plastic bowl (you can usually buy milk at the airport)
Leftover Food from home (potato salad, egg salad, quinoa, rice dish, etc.)

I also suggest that you carry a letter from your doctor that states you are on a medical diet and it is common for you to carry food with you onto the plane. I've had my individual-size peanut butter containers taken away more than once, going through the security line.

If I do not have access to a grocery store in my destination city, I always buy a couple of days' worth of fruit in the airport where I land. Having fruit on hand certainly helps out with some breakfasts and snacks during the day.

Tip #4—Research Your Destination City

Contact celiac support groups. Your gluten-free travel plans should start weeks before you leave home. It's really easy to contact the local celiac support group in your destination city. People are usually very willing to help you with local knowledge of grocery stores and restaurants. They can also advise you on gluten-free bakeries in the area.

Contact grocery stores. Contact the grocery stores in your destination city. The store managers will usually provide a list of gluten-free products in their store. For example, I always find out if they carry a brand of gluten-free cereal that I like so I don't have to pack the cereal in my suitcase. You may have access to different gluten-free brands and manufacturers in that area of the country. Please keep in mind that products that have recently removed their "gluten-free" label and replaced it with "made with no gluten ingredients" may not be testing their ingredient suppliers or end product for gluten. Cross-contamination may be an issue.

Contact restaurant managers/chefs. Try to get a personal recommendation for a contact at local restaurants. A "transfer of trust" from a local celiac is extremely valuable. You'll find that if the local celiacs trust a restaurant and manager, then all you need is a brief conversation with the manager. Always call during nonbusy hours a couple of days before your arrival, to verify their comfort level with preparing gluten-free options. Obviously, larger metropolitan areas such as New York and Denver are more gluten-free-friendly. For example, I have found an Italian restaurant in Denver called Abrusci's (www.abruscis .com); Steve Progar, the owner, has a friend who is celiac and he has developed a gluten-free menu that rivals the regular menu in quantity and quality.

Tip #5—Develop a Hotel Strategy

There are various options and levels of hotels that offer a suite or kitchen setup inside the hotel room to facilitate easier eating. Most of the Marriott and Hilton chain of hotels offer a refrigerator and microwave oven in your room. I've also been in situations where the front desk will reserve a refrigerator for your room at no extra charge if you are on a medical diet. It never hurts to ask questions, as I have even heard of hotels where guests can leave their special diets in the staff refrigerator!

Research the grocery stores near the hotels that you are considering. It's easy to be within walking distance of a store that has fresh food or possibly gluten-free food as an option.

Some brands of dishwashing detergent (such as Palmolive) manufacture individual cloths that are sold in plastic containers. When you wet the single-serving cloth, you have plenty of suds to clean your utensils, electric teakettle, plate, or bowl. All you have to do is just throw the cloth away when you're done. This solution is perfect for hotel rooms.

Tip #6—Understand Your Infrastructure Needs

If you are traveling by car and you plan to eat some of your meals in your hotel room, then there is a subset of supplies that is needed for your journey. Check to see if your hotel has any of these items available and ask beforehand about the hotel rules as to cooking on their property.

- Microwavable plate, cup, bowl
- Plastic silverware or a set of metal camping utensils
- A manual can opener
- Electric teakettle or fondue pot
- George Forman or equivalent electric grill
- Napkins, wet wipes
- Plastic bags, plastic wrap, aluminum foil

Carrying a cooler in the car is also an easy way to ensure that you have safe food with you at all times. Convenience stores, gas stations, and/or grocery stores often have microwave ovens that the employees may let you use to heat your food. Some grocery stores and natural food stores that have an eating area may have a microwave oven available as well.

Tip #7—Be Prepared

Cook at home. It's important to take advantage of your kitchen at home by cooking or baking before you leave your house. I usually make corn on the cob, quinoa, and gluten-free cookies before I leave. Quinoa is good cold, warm, or hot. I'll also freeze my cookies so they last longer during travel. It's nice to have a variety of food with you at all times. Think through what else you can make for dinner and have as leftovers on the road. Cook extra quantities and freeze them in portion sizes to take on your trip.

Travel cards. There are various travel or cook cards in many languages that you can carry with you to different restaurants in different countries. These can be extremely useful, particularly when you are not fluent in the local language. Be mindful of the fact that cross-contamination may still occur, so do not be embarrassed to explain in detail how your food must be prepared safely.

Tip #8—Balance Is Key

Variety is the spice of life. Remember that you will get very bored eating the same cereal and meal solutions every day. Think through how many days you are traveling and what your grocery store and restaurant options will be throughout your travel. I learned this lesson when I was once in a city where I could find only one restaurant that could make only one gluten-free meal—I ate that meal every other night for dinner. Although I was grateful for a gluten-free option, having only one choice made my mealtime very boring after only a few short days.

It is no fun to rely solely on packing your own meals if you have the option of eating safely at a restaurant once in awhile during your travels. Be sure, though, that if you are traveling with someone other than your spouse or close family members (who already understand your food requirements), you communicate details in advance of what traveling with you entails. My husband and I were recently attending a conference with some friends for a week. Even though they all knew I had celiac disease, at restaurants they were sometimes still shocked by my eating habits. In some restaurants I would eat food I had brought myself, and in other restaurants where I had already had discussions with the manager, there was still the "drama" of walking the waitstaff through the gluten-free instructions. It's important to prepare whomever you're traveling with, to reduce stress or anxiety when dining out.

Don't forget your vitamins and supplements on your trip. As you know, many processed gluten-free foods don't have the added nutrients you need.

So, ensure that you are taking enough vitamins to supplement your diet. Extra fruits and vegetables are easy to add into your diet.

It's also important to get some exercise while you're on the road. Climb the hotel stairs, go for a walk, or work out in the hotel's fitness room.

◇ ◇ ◇

IN A SENTENCE

> *Unwinding and relaxing when you travel means knowing where you're going, how you're getting there, and planning your meals accordingly; invest the time to research trip-specific challenges and their solutions, so you don't spend any of your travel time worrying about safe meals!*

MONTH **12**

What If You Don't Feel Better Yet?

ARGUABLY, THE hardest part about adapting to a gluten-free lifestyle is managing the expectation that it will miraculously and immediately solve all of your health problems, only to find that it hasn't. As you have learned, everyone's system rebounds and heals at different rates, largely depending on how long celiac symptoms went undetected or improperly diagnosed. For adults, it can take as long as two years for intestinal villi to completely heal. Other factors may be at work, though, and need to be considered if your symptoms have not resolved.

This month, we'll look at possible sources of hidden gluten contamination and other health factors that can affect your symptoms.

Pharmaceuticals and Over-the-Counter Medications

One of the most overlooked sources of gluten is often our medications. The inactive ingredients, or excipients, which often make up the bulk of **prescription and over-the-counter (OTC) medications** are regulated by the Food and Drug Administration (FDA) for product safety, but the FDA does not specifically regulate the quality or type of filler a pharmaceutical company may use. These fillers are the primary source of any possible gluten contamination in medicines, so it is important to understand their sources and functions, to protect yourself.

The inactive ingredients added to medicines may be used as lubricants, to provide shape and bulk, or to absorb water (which causes the tablet to swell and disintegrate). Starches are often the substances used for these functions. As with food products, starches may be derived from multiple sources: corn, potato, rice, tapioca, or wheat (barley and rye are not used in medications). Unlike food products or even nutritional supplements, prescription and OTC medications using these starchy fillers are not required to include labeling specifically designating their origins. Pharmaceutical companies have not historically concerned themselves with these raw materials, other than to know whether they are safe and that they perform the required task in the medication. Pharmaceutical manufacturers obtain the starches from outside suppliers and that is sometimes all they know about the ingredient.

Inactive Ingredient Labels on Your Medicines [1]

Cellulose	obtained from fibrous plant material = gluten-free
Dextrans	sugar derived from corn- and potato starch = gluten-free
Dextrates	sugar that may be derived from wheat–call manufacturer
Dextri-maltose	sugar that may be derived from barley–call manufacturer
Dextrins	may be derived from wheat–call manufacturer
Dextrose	sugar derived from cornstarch = gluten-free
Glycerin	usually derived from petroleum = gluten-free
Lactose	milk sugar = gluten-free
Pregelatinized starch	may be derived from wheat–call manufacturer
Purified alcohol	contains no protein = gluten-free
Sodium starch glycolate	may be derived from wheat–call manufacturer
Starch	may be derived from wheat–call manufacturer
Stearates	a fat = gluten-free
Sucrose	refined sugar = gluten-free

1. Steven Plogsted, "Medications and Celiac Disease—Tips from a Pharmacist," *Practical Gastroenterology* (January 2007): 58–64, The Celiac Diet, Series #5, Carol Rees Parrish, ed.

So how do you determine if your medication is indeed gluten-free? The best and only real answer is to contact the manufacturer yourself. Often the FAQ page of a pharmaceutical Web site will have the information you need. If you are more comfortable calling, though, you can usually find the phone number you will need on the packaging or product insert; otherwise, your pharmacist is your best resource. Always inform your pharmacist—every time you have a prescription filled—that you have celiac disease and cannot take any medications containing gluten. Take over-the-counter medications to the pharmacy window and seek their help in confirming whether the products are gluten-free. Together, you should be able to find the answer.

Some particularly helpful free resources can also help you learn more about glutens in your medicines. One maintained and periodically updated by a clinical pharmacist is www.GlutenFreeDrugs.com. Another with free and paid information is www.clanthompson.com.

As with foods, you need to be vigilant about rechecking the gluten-free status of your medications whenever there is any reformulation of the product, or if you have gone back to a medication you used to take. It is also a good practice to ask your prescribing physician for first- and second-choice medications, in the event that the first choice prescription contains gluten. Also, have your physician indicate that generic formulations are optional, but not required, so that the pharmacist is free to fill the drug formulation that is gluten-free. On the other hand, ask your physician to note "dispense as written" for brand-name drugs you know to be gluten-free, so as to assure that a particular formulation is filled for a patient. Sometimes a name-brand drug is gluten-free, but the generic version is not, or vice versa—it is always good to have a backup plan before you spend hours waiting for the pharmacy to confirm changes to the prescription with your physician. You may have to fight with your insurance company for coverage of a nongeneric medication, so arm yourself at the pharmacy with all the information you need, to prove that you had no other gluten-free choice.[2]

In summary, medications are an extremely plausible source of gluten contamination. If you are continuing to suffer from painful or unpleasant physical symptoms, check your existing medicines—prescription and over-the-counter—

---

2. Nancy Lapid, "Celiac Disease: How to Protect Yourself from Hidden Gluten in Medications," About.com, Inc., part of the New York Times Company, http://celiacdisease.about.com/od/medicalguidelines/a/medications.htm (February 14, 2008).

to be sure that you are not unwittingly ingesting gluten. Keep a watchful eye out and enlist your pharmacist's assistance to prevent yourself from taking the wrong medicines in the future.

Religious Practices

In examining your habits and eating practices in search of possible gluten contamination, take a look at periodic possibilities. These occasions will present themselves most often outside of the home and may occur in situations where you feel you have no control. One of these circumstances is in various religious rites.

The Jewish festival of Passover (Pesach) often causes confusion and fear of obligatory contamination for those with celiac disease. Jews observe Passover in part by eating unleavened bread for the seven-day festival, celebrating both the fact that the Jews were spared (or passed over) when God slayed the firstborn sons in Egypt and the subsequent exodus of Jews from Egypt after having suffered generations of slavery. The Jews left in such great haste that their bread did not have time to rise. Hence, celebrations of Passover have revolved around the obligation to eat matzo, or unleavened bread, during this time. Matzo is traditionally made from wheat or other gluten-containing grains, but Jewish law does not require that matzo contain wheat or gluten.[3] Gluten-free matzo is now commercially manufactured, mostly using oat flour, and recipes are available to make your own unleavened matzo during Passover.

Unlike the Jewish traditions, the Catholic rite of Holy Eucharist does require the Host to contain wheat, and Hosts that have no gluten are considered invalid for Mass. In many churches, this ceremony occurs every week during the church service and has generated great spiritual and ethical controversy.

The Catholic Church has maintained the belief throughout the centuries that Jesus used a wheat bread at the Last Supper. Despite health concerns by celiacs and others, the Church has not wavered on the position that celebration of the Holy Eucharist must still be done with wheat. In fact, then Cardinal Joseph Ratzinger (now Pope Benedict XVI) officially reiterated that

---

3. Rabbi Avraham Juravel, "Gluten Intolerance, Celiac, Allergies and Pesach," Orthodox Union, http://www.oukosher.org/index.php/passover/article/7565/.

position when he wrote to the Presidents of Episcopal Conferences in 2003. At that time, though, he offered two acceptable solutions to this dilemma: that celiacs and others who are intolerant of gluten may, through the doctrine of concomitance, receive full communion by only taking consecrated wine; or that an approved low-gluten Host may be used in the alternative.[4]

The latter solution was only accepted after over a decade of dedicated experimentation by the Benedictine Sisters of Perpetual Adoration of Clyde, Missouri. These nuns are the largest religious producers of Communion wafers, shipping over 2 million wafers a week—many of those of the low-gluten variety. According to research on the gluten content of these handmade wheat starch wafers, this Host has a 0.01 percent gluten content—enough to qualify as valid for Catholic Communion, but not enough to jeopardize the health of celiacs. Extrapolated out into micrograms, the Host the sisters produce would enable a celiac to eat up to 270 wafers per day to reach the scientifically accepted "danger point" for those with celiac disease.[5]

Despite these apparent concessions, parents and children seeking to participate in the rite of the Holy Eucharist in the Catholic Church worldwide have repeatedly been faced with difficult choices, feelings of isolation, belief that they have been forsaken, and concerns that they are being treated as second-class Catholics. News reports appear regularly around the world documenting how individuals with celiac disease are denied the opportunity to commune in the Catholic Church.[6]

Other Christian faiths do allow nonglutenous, non-wheat-based Communion wafers, believing less in the importance of the chemical makeup of the Host than in the significance of the sign itself. Most Protestant faiths allow rice-based or other non-gluten-containing Communion wafers, so it is worth investigating options with your own church. The risk of contamination due to intinction (others' dipping their glutenous communion wafers into the chalice of wine, thus contaminating the wine with gluten) is still present, so assigning a particular chalice to gluten-free participants, or at

---

4. United States Conference of Catholic Bishops, "The Use of Mustum and Low-Gluten Hosts at Mass," Secretariat for Divine Worship, http://www.usccb.org/litergy/innews/1103.shtml.

5. Benedictine Sisters, "Low Gluten Altar Breads: The Work of Our Hands," Benedictine Sisters of Perpetual Adoration, http://benedictinesisters.org/bread/low_gluten.php.

6. See, for instance, ThinkSpain, Religion, "Church Denies Gluten-Free Communion Wafer Option to Coeliac Sufferer," March 12, 2008, http://www.thinkspain.com/news-spain/14645/church-denies-gluten-free-communion-wafer-option-to-coeliac-sufferer.

minimum, ensuring that you are at the front of the Communion line, are safe practices you should consider.[7]

Non-Celiac-Related Health Problems

You have now spent twelve months learning about, tasting, cooking, and generally perseverating over a gluten-free diet. Until it becomes totally second nature to you, this level of worry is somewhat natural. The tendency is to attribute any continuing or future gastrointestinal distress to unmitigated celiac disease and gluten contamination. While an examination of possible gluten sources in your diet and lifestyle is useful, you should also remain aware that your body remains susceptible to the same environmental exposures as every other person's. In addition, depending on how long you manifested active, untreated celiac disease, your age at diagnosis, any other physical conditions, and your own unique physiology, you may suffer more severely or for a longer duration from additional symptoms that have no direct correlation to celiac disease. Often, for example, newly diagnosed celiacs have difficulty digesting very fatty foods until the small intestine has had sufficient time to heal. Discuss these concerns with your doctor as you regularly follow-up through the months and years ahead.

Consider that you may have other food allergies or intolerances, and reexamine your diet for triggers to your symptoms.[8] Some folks feel negative effects from some kinds of gluten-free flours, such as bean or nut flours. Experiment with eliminating certain other foods like these from your diet one at a time, to see if you feel any difference over a period of weeks. If you do notice a change, gradually reintroduce one food at a time to see if you can hone in on the exact trigger. You may also want to have separate food allergy testing done through an allergist. Many of these tests are done through blood work and do not involve a great deal of time or stress to your body.

Another consideration is whether you have been exposed to a virus or bacteria that has caused the symptoms you have. Perhaps you have been on antibiotics that upset the delicate balance of your intestinal flora. Antibiotics themselves may also cause their own negative side effects. All of these questions

---

7. June Marcley, "Wheat-Free Worship: The Communion Conundrum," *Living Without* magazine, http://www.livingwithout.com/features/feature-wheatfreeworship.html.

8. The Children's Health and Nutrition Foundation, *Celiac Disease*, http://celiachealth.org/.

should help you to identify whether there is another factor at work causing your physical distress.

One of the most common causes of some amount of gastrointestinal symptoms in celiacs, despite following a rigorous gluten-free diet, is **lactose intolerance**. A large percentage of diagnosed celiacs are lactose intolerant for at least some period of time following implementation of a gluten-free diet. Incidentally, this works both ways, as a large percentage of those who are lactose intolerant are also celiac.[9]

Thinking back to the first week, you may recall the condition of villous atrophy and all of its many stages. **Lactase enzymes** are necessary to break down the lactose—or milk sugar—in dairy products, and these enzymes are uniquely generated on the tips of the villi that line the intestinal tract. If the villi are blunted or damaged completely, it makes sense that the tips of these villi would be the first to go and the last to come back when the villi regenerate under healthy (nongluten) conditions. Depending again on your unique physiology and on the length of time between villous atrophy and implementation of a gluten-free diet, the villi might not ever fully regenerate and the lactase enzyme-producing tips would be the first casualties. Some of us (myself, unfortunately, included) never shake this condition and are forced to either avoid dairy entirely or to reduce dairy intake and use lactase enzyme supplements as needed to control symptoms.

Incidence

○ Secondary lactase deficiency is estimated to be 20–40%

○ Increasing lactose intolerance with prolongation of arriving at CD diagnosis

○ Increased incidence in patients with GI symptoms in CD

○ Decreased calcium and Vitamin D intake in Lactose intolerance

Treatment

○ Gluten-free diet

○ Temporary lactose-reduction

○ Lactase enzymes

○ Gluten-free, lactose-free milk

○ Gluten-free milk substitute

○ Supplement with gluten-free calcium and Vitamin D where appropriate

---

9. Scott Adams, "Celiac Disease Common in Patients with Lactose Intolerance," Celiac.com (March 30, 2005), http://www.celiac.com.

Unlike celiac disease, lactose intolerance bears no long-term negative effects other than sometimes painful and embarrassing gastrointestinal symptoms such as abdominal pain or distention, diarrhea, or gas. As with gluten or wheat intolerance, these symptoms are relieved when the lactose leaves your system (try to avoid taking antidiarrheal remedies that will only prolong how long the lactose stays in your system) and will not cause permanent damage. Your approach to lactose intolerance therefore should be with whatever actions you are most comfortable.

Other Possible (Nonceliac) Offending Causes for Gastrointestinal Distress

acidic foods

antibiotics

food allergies (especially to milk protein [casein], soy, nuts, eggs, and corn)

guar gum

intolerances to gluten-free flours (particularly bean or nut flours)

lactose intolerance

Olestra

other food intolerances

intolerances to nonorganic substances used to grow, process, or preserve foods

sorbitol (nondigestible sugar found in some medication and dietetic candy)

viruses and bacterial infections

IN A SENTENCE

Exposure to hidden sources of gluten, non-gluten-related health problems, and food allergies or intolerances may affect the pace or completeness of your total recovery.

living

Looking Back and Looking Forward

THIS POINT should be one for self-congratulation as much as for anything else. Look how far you have come! Remember all the horrible fears you had about living gluten-free, or the negative things people may have told you, and appreciate how wrong they were and the value of a positive attitude. You could have let their predictions and anxieties become your own, but you didn't. You made the choice to instead delve further into the opportunities your diagnosis has offered you and how it can improve your life on so many levels.

In the years to come, you will continue to learn more about celiac disease and living gluten-free, but your learning curve now will be easy by comparison. Stay the course and enjoy the ride from now on, and you will live happier and healthier knowing you are in more control of your health destiny. I wish you all the best in your new gluten-free life; may your respect for your body and your life be infectious in helping others to similarly embrace the opportunities this diagnosis presents to them.

I leave you with the words of Annella McLaughlin, a celiac mother and wife whom I have come to know only through her overt positive attitude and gratitude for the new life that she has seized for herself and her family. Celiacs like Annella are an inspiration for us all and a reminder that life is truly what we make it.

◇ ◇ ◇

Annella McLaughlin's Story

When I consider all I have learned and experienced in the twelve months since being diagnosed with celiac disease, my previous gluten-filled diet feels like a lifetime ago. Although I felt quite ill at the time and was anxious for a medical explanation, finding out I had celiac was more than I expected to hear.

I met with a dietitian shortly after being diagnosed, and when the restrictions of a gluten-free diet were explained to me, I was honestly brought to tears. The information I was given had such a negative spin to it, I felt devastated. I was told, "Good luck being able to eat out in a restaurant again," and "You can find a few gluten-free items in our local grocery stores, but not many."

I began to mentally run through the short list of meals I felt competent in preparing at home and realized all were laden with gluten. I then reflected on the many nights my husband and I resorted to take-out dinner due to our busy schedules and knew those, too, were no longer an option. I felt sheer panic as I tried to think of anything I knew how to make that was naturally gluten-free. The kitchen has never been a comfortable place for me and cooking dinner "from scratch" translated into opening various boxes and cans of processed foods and adding meat or pasta to finish off the dish. To say I was overwhelmed would have been an understatement. I truly wondered if I was going to starve.

At that point I allowed myself a couple of days of self-pity and shed more than a few tears. I then made a decision. I was not going to allow my diagnosis of celiac to define me or my life in a negative way. I was going to have to step up to the challenge and learn how to prepare safe and delicious foods for myself and my family. I was going to have to begin an entirely new lifestyle.

My supportive husband agreed with my decision to make our dinners gluten-free for the entire family, and I searched the Internet for cookbooks that weren't too intimidating to my novice cooking skills, but also contained recipes that sounded enjoyable for our tastes. It didn't take me long to find Jules Shepard's book: *Nearly Normal Cooking for Gluten-Free Eating*. When I received the book and read her introduction I knew I had found my cooking guide. I felt like I had invited a dear friend into my home and she had expressed exactly what I had been feeling and thinking about celiac. Yes, there were far worse things a person could have to deal with, but living gluten-free is not easy. My catchphrase about living with celiac is: "It's doable . . . very challenging . . . but doable."

The biggest challenge for me in living this new lifestyle has been having to plan meals in advance and develop my cooking skills to be able to prepare them. I realized very quickly that if I wanted to be able to eat, I would have to have meals and snacks outlined and available long before my hunger strikes. I was initially carrying around a bag of carrots, rice cakes, and a small jar of peanut butter. I am now happy to report that I haven't eaten a rice cake in months . . . and I thought they were going to be a staple for me!

Planning meals is something I have never mastered in the past, and the concept of having dinner prepared when my husband came home from work was completely foreign to me. However, because of my celiac condition, I am now doing both. Because of my gluten-free lifestyle, my family is enjoying better meals than we ever did before and I have my diagnosis of celiac disease to thank.

I have three children under the age of eight and one is a very picky eater. Despite my trepidation, I dusted off our family dinner table and turned to Jules's cookbook to start preparing gluten-free meals. I could not believe the pure joy I felt each time I served a home-cooked, gluten-free meal my kids ate without complaint and my husband enjoyed with many compliments. Everything I tried from the cookbook was a success, even with my inexperience! I am still shocked that my husband and children request "Mom's" brownies or muffins. My son even asked me to make gluten-free brownies for his birthday dessert, and he doesn't even have celiac disease!

Celiac disease has brought my family to the dinner table, *together*. We sit down every evening and enjoy well-balanced, gluten-free meals from my kitchen. Of course there are times I miss the freedom of being able to pick up a quick dinner on a busy evening, but I have come up with my own time-crunch menus. I had hoped I would find the positive in my diagnosis, and I can honestly say I have: I can cook dinner for my family! I prepare delicious food that is safe for my gluten-free lifestyle and no one misses out on the flavor. I even hosted Thanksgiving dinner and Christmas morning breakfast this year for a small group of extended family—both prepared gluten-free. It is shocking to me what I have been able to accomplish!

I certainly don't want to give the impression that living gluten-free has been sunshine and roses. There are many challenges I have yet to master. Social events are uncomfortable for me, as most revolve around food. Vacation travel requires far more planning than ever before. I have had to spend time researching restaurants and stores at our vacation destinations so I can have the peace of mind of knowing I will be able to eat without packing my entire fridge, freezer, and pantry. We have chosen to arrange for accommodations that are equipped with a kitchen. This proves to be convenient for my dietary needs as well as offering more choices for my young family. In my home town, only a couple of restaurants offer gluten-free menus, so those are the places my husband and I go each week for our date night. I am thankful to have the option of a safe restaurant-prepared meal.

Looking back over the months since my diagnosis I am happy to say my life has actually improved immensely. My husband has told many people he is eating better than he has in our past seventeen years of marriage. My children are well versed on celiac disease and are happy to consume my home-made dishes. My health has improved, and accomplishing that through dietary changes has given me a sense of accomplishment. I am grateful to be living a lifestyle that is not only safe for me but truly a blessing for my family. That is the message I would like to share with anyone who has recently been diagnosed. Eating gluten-free may seem impossible and extremely restrictive, but it is doable and can even be enjoyed. Most important, it can bring your family closer together.

◇ ◇ ◇

IN A SENTENCE

> *Living with celiac disease and living gluten-free are adjustments you probably didn't count on in your life plan; however, now that you understand the gift of good health you have been given by being able to largely control your future health through diet, and you have learned how to make your favorite foods again safely, there is no reason to ever look back.*

Glossary

AUTOIMMUNE DISEASE is a condition in which the body attacks *itself* in an inappropriate immune system reaction to a perceived body invader.

BANANA DIET was the only prescribed treatment course for celiac disease during the early to mid-twentieth century. This diet was primarily comprised of bananas, and patients were instructed to follow this diet exclusively for a number of years, until they were "cured" of celiac disease. Fortunately, gluten has since been discovered as the true trigger for celiac disease; therefore, a gluten-free diet is now the lifelong treatment for those diagnosed with celiac disease.

CELIAC ICEBERG describes the phenomenon that the majority of those with undiagnosed celiac disease actually suffer no overt symptoms, even though they still risk suffering its complications.

CELIAC PANEL refers to the blood tests used to discern whether an individual carries a higher-than-normal level of certain antibodies in his or her blood that would indicate that the person's body is exhibiting a celiac autoimmune reaction. This panel typically includes tests for anti-endomysial antibody (IgA), antitissue transglutaminase (IgA), anti-gliadin (IgA and IgG), and total serum IgA against particular antigens in the small bowel like tissue transglutaminase (tTG).

CELIAC SPRUE (celiac/cœliac disease, nontropical sprue, or gluten-sensitive enteropathy) is a hereditary autoimmune disease that manifests in a chronic and permanent sensitivity to the food protein gluten, found in the grains wheat, barley, and rye. Individuals with active celiac disease may exhibit intestinal or extraintestinal symptoms, making it often difficult to diagnose without appropriate diagnostic blood tests and an intestinal endoscopy.

COOK CARDS are small cards carried with you to a restaurant or while traveling, to clearly define and indicate in translated languages what food restrictions are necessary when preparing your food. These can be taken back to the chef, given to the manager, or used to question the waiter about the menu ingredients and are a key component to eating out safely with celiac disease.

DERMATITIS HERPETIFORMIS (DH) is an itchy, blistering, and painful skin rash (usually around the elbows, knees, and buttocks), which is another manifestation of celiac disease.

ENDOSCOPIC BIOPSY is a minimally invasive surgical procedure whereby a small tube is inserted via the mouth of a sedated individual and passes into the upper intestinal tract to provide for visual inspection and biopsy of tissue for diagnostic purposes.

FOOD ALLERGEN LABELING AND CONSUMER PROTECTION ACT (FALCPA) of 2004 (U.S.) requires that manufacturers must list on a product label any of the eight main food allergens (milk, egg, peanuts, tree nuts, fish, shellfish, soy, and wheat) if they are contained in that manufactured product or if they are secondary ingredients to the spices, natural or artificial flavorings, additives, or colorings. The law covers food products, dietary supplements, and vitamins, but it does not apply to over-the-counter medications or to prescription drugs.

FOOD ALLERGIES occur in individuals whose bodies are intolerant to certain foods to such a degree that a histamine reaction occurs relatively soon after ingestion. These reactions are not autoimmune in nature, can be life-threatening in those with severe allergic reactions, and do not cause long-term damage to the intestinal tract.

FOOD LABELING in the United States is controlled by the FDA (Food and Drug Administration). Recently the FDA has propounded certain labeling requirements for foods whose manufacturers claim to be "gluten-free." This standard will allow the term *gluten-free* to be used on labels indicating the food is free of the following: any of the prohibited grains of wheat, barley, rye, or their hybrids; ingredients derived from these prohibited grains and that still contain gluten; and any ingredients that contain more than twenty parts per million (ppm) of gluten per gram of food.

GLIADIN is the specific component of the food protein gluten that is contained in wheat, barley, and rye. Gliadin is the catalyst for the inappropriate autoimmune reaction known as celiac disease.

GLUTEN is a protein molecule contained in the grains wheat, barley, and rye. It provides elasticity in baking; without gluten, substitutes such as xanthan or guar gums will provide the elasticity needed to hold baked goods together.

GLUTEN INTOLERANCE manifests with many of the same overt symptoms as celiac disease, but testing for celiac disease by bloodwork and endoscopy is negative. Those with gluten intolerance learn through trial and error that gluten is the culprit for their uncomfortable symptoms and, once they adopt a gluten-free diet, live an otherwise normal healthy life.

HIPAA (HEALTH INSURANCE PORTABILITY AND ACCOUNTABILITY ACT OF 1996) (U.S.) is a federal law that was enacted to protect patients' rights in certain health insurance matters, including limiting insurance exclusions for preexisting conditions.

HLA TYPING is the genetic testing used to determine if a person carries DQ2 and DQ8—two genes found in nearly every person with celiac disease. If you do not carry this HLA typing, it is highly unlikely that you have or will ever develop celiac disease.

IMPAIRED FECUNDITY means that a person is not surgically sterile yet it is nonetheless difficult or impossible for that person to get pregnant or to carry a pregnancy to term.

INFERTILE means that a person is not surgically sterile, has not used contraception in the past twelve months, but has not become pregnant.

IRRITABLE BOWEL SYNDROME (IBS) describes a group of symptoms, including abdominal pain or discomfort caused by cramping, bloating, gas, constipation, and/or diarrhea. IBS affects the colon, or large bowel, as opposed to celiac disease, which affects the small intestine.

LACTASE ENZYMES are generated in the villi lining the intestinal tract and are necessary to break down the lactose in ingested dairy products. Lactase enzymes are also available in supplement form for those who are lactose intolerant and wish to still enjoy dairy products.

LACTOSE INTOLERANCE is a condition whereby the body lacks the lactase enzymes necessary to break down the milk sugar (lactose) in dairy products when they are eaten. Resulting symptoms typically include intestinal cramping, gas, bloating, and diarrhea.

MALABSORPTION is the condition whereby the body ineffectively absorbs nutrients from ingested food, leading to such conditions as gas, diarrhea, and ultimately to malnutrition.

OATS were a grain originally thought to contain gluten and therefore included in the list of grains to avoid on a gluten-free diet. However, recent studies have shown that oats are inherently gluten-free and therefore are acceptable to most celiacs, so long as they are grown, milled, and processed in a strictly controlled gluten-free environment.

PREEXISTING CONDITIONS that can limit health insurance coverage under HIPPA are limited to conditions whereby medical advice, diagnosis, or treatment was either recommended or received within the six-month period before an insurance enrollment or coverage date.

VILLI are fingerlike tissue projections that line the upper intestinal tract and generate enzymes to break down food as well as absorb food components for healthy digestion.

VILLOUS ATROPHY is the condition whereby the villi become blunted and eventually flattened due to repeated absorption of gluten by a person with celiac disease. This condition ultimately leads to malabsorption and malnutrition.

ZONULIN is an intestinal protein that regulates intestinal permeability. In those with celiac disease, gluten exposure causes an increase in zonulin production, thereby increasing their intestinal permeability to the point of actual leakage between the intestines and other body compartments.

Frequently Asked Questions

Q: How often should I have a checkup with my doctor?

A: Initially, you want to follow up with your gastroenterologist at regular intervals coinciding with bloodwork that he or she prescribes. You will eventually scale back to once every six months and then once a year if you are doing well and are confident on the gluten-free diet. Of course, your physician is going to recommend a course of treatment and examinations specific to your needs, so you need to adhere to his or her recommendations, which may differ from this model. As a general rule, once you are stabilized on a gluten-free diet, celiac serology should be repeated every year or so to be sure that you are not continuing to have problems—silent or overt—with celiac disease.

Q: How long will it take for me to feel better once I start a gluten-free diet?

A: Just as everyone has a unique set of symptoms resulting from celiac disease, everyone recovers from gluten damage at different rates. You will likely feel somewhat better within days of starting a strict gluten-free diet, although it can take three to six months for younger people and up to two years for older adults to have completely healed intestinal villi once more. Be patient and, most important, remain true to the gluten-free diet; you will heal and you will feel better if you keep to the diet.

Q: If I have celiac disease, should I have my children checked for celiac disease?

A: If you have a confirmed diagnosis of celiac disease, you should speak with your doctor and with your children's pediatrician regarding their recommendations. If your children have no overt symptoms of CD, your pediatrician will likely recommend running the celiac serology the next time each child has other bloodwork done and then every two years or so thereafter. Your children will probably continue to eat gluten to some degree, despite your diet, so they will more than likely test positive for celiac if they are in active stages of the disease. You may choose instead to have them each tested by doing DNA tests to look for specific celiac markers. If they do not have the recognized markers for celiac, it is highly unlikely (if not impossible) that they will ever contract CD, thus eliminating the need to ever repeat the celiac bloodwork panel. Other first-degree relatives, in particular, should consider following the same course to test for celiac disease.

Q: Should I be taking additional vitamins now that I have celiac disease?

A: If you had nutrient deficiencies as a result of active celiac disease, your physician or nutritionist will likely encourage you to take some nutritional supplements in addition to a high-quality multivitamin. Some of the kinds of nutrients you may want to supplement are vitamins B_{12}, B_6, K, and E. Folic acid and calcium are two additional supplements that many celiacs should consider adding to their vitamin regimen. Depending on your symptoms, you may also find that probiotics are beneficial for you. Make sure you check with your pharmacist if you are at all unclear from the labels of any of these products whether they are gluten-free, and always ask your doctor's advice on any supplementation.

Q: Is it really a big deal if I "cheat" once in awhile and have gluten?

A: Even if you do not feel direct effects from eating gluten, if you have celiac disease, rest assured that your body is suffering effects from exposure. Research has shown that any amount of gluten can damage the intestinal villi of a person with celiac disease (even as little as 1/8 teaspoon of gluten—approximately 1/1000 of a slice of bread). Even without symptoms, you are still risking medical complications from CD if you do not follow a strict gluten-free diet.[1] Given the volume and variety of wonderful foods you can safely consume without causing harm, there is really no reason to "cheat" and endanger your future health.

Q: What happens if I unknowingly eat something containing gluten?

A: Celiac disease is an autoimmune disorder, not an allergy. Therefore, you may or may not feel physical effects from contamination. You should treat any symptoms as best you can, eat easily digestible gluten-free foods until you feel better, and learn from any inadvertent mistakes that you may have made this time. Most important, do not blame yourself; move on and know that you will feel better soon if you continue to eat gluten-free.

---

1. Healthlink, "Celiac Disease," Medical College of Wisconsin, http://healthlink.mcw.edu/article/956622658.html.

Q: **In a nutshell, how do I go out to eat again safely?**

A: Carry and use a "cook card" like that found on page 120. You must be comfortable and confident asking questions at the restaurant, in advance when possible, and again when you arrive. Ask politely to speak with the manager, owner, or chef and, at least initially, do not bother with chain restaurants unless they have a preprinted gluten-free menu and the staff seems to understand the severity of your restrictions and cross-contamination. A good rule of thumb is to order foods without sauces or dressings and stick with steamed vegetables and rice. As you become accustomed to menus and eating out gluten-free, you will find restaurants and dishes that you enjoy that are more exciting and are still safe.

Q: **How do I bake my favorite foods again, but bake them gluten-free?**

A: This question may seem tough at first, but once you find a good, truly all-purpose gluten-free flour mix, you can jump right back into the kitchen and begin your own experiments with your favorite recipes. Most gluten-free baked goods need a bit of extra leavening (e.g., baking soda and/or baking powder) and perhaps extra moisture, since gluten-free flours tend to absorb moisture more quickly than traditional wheat flours. Initially you should buy a premade flour so that you can get started right away enjoying good gluten-free food. Later, you may want to try recipes to make your own flour (my recipe is given on page 48).

Q: **How do I store gluten-free flour?**

A: Unless you are keeping a lot of high-fat gluten-free flours, you should be able to store your flours in airtight containers in cool, dark locations. Check the expiration dates on the flours when you purchase them; the dates should give you a proper indication of how long they will keep under these conditions. Other higher-fat flours, such as nut, bean, and whole-grain flours, may need to be kept in the refrigerator or freezer if you plan on keeping them for a while.

Q: **What is the best way to get the elasticity back in gluten-free foods?**

A: The ingredients most often used to create glutenlike elasticity in gluten-free baking are xanthan gum and guar gum. These are typically well tolerated by celiacs and are available at health and organic food stores and online. An all-purpose gluten-free flour should already have one of these ingredients included; if it does not, pick another flour. These gums are the most expensive ingredient in any gluten-free all-purpose flour, so make sure it is already included before you choose a brand.

Q: **What are the best, most useful, and most versatile gluten-free flours to have in my cupboard?**

A: I have found that in addition to an all-purpose gluten-free flour mix, cornstarch, potato starch, tapioca starch, and white rice flour are the most often used in my house. I like these flours because they have the least distinctive taste, so they are very versatile and are equally good in a roux as in a muffin. They are also very widely available and fairly cheap, as gluten-free flours go. I enjoy experimenting with some other flours for additional nutritional and taste variation, and in my consulting work I often use more unusual flours to meet the needs of individuals with other food restrictions. Some that I particularly enjoy are amaranth flour, almond flour, buckwheat flour, brown rice flour, coconut flour, and flaxseed meal. I have tried nearly every gluten-free flour available, and most are good, but only in certain recipes. If you have extra time, energy, money, and cabinet space to invest in lots of other gluten-free flours, go to town! Just understand that some of the higher-fat flours may need to be refrigerated or frozen to store them for any length of time.

Q: **What are the most essential ingredients to have on hand for living gluten-free?**

A: You should be sure to have plenty of gluten-free munchies and snacking material: fresh fruit, pretzels, popcorn, protein bars, chips, yogurt—whatever you enjoy to get you between meals. Of course, you will also want to have either the ingredients to make, or have a premixed all-purpose gluten-free flour. Then, you should choose a few meals you would like to make every week or so, and have those ingredients on your regular shopping list: rice; gluten-free pasta; pasta sauce; fresh vegetables; fresh meat, chicken, or fish; salad ingredients; ice cream; applesauce; and the like. If you enjoy particular types of foods such as salads, be sure to have a good gluten-free dressing in your refrigerator. If you really like Asian foods, seek out a gluten-free soy sauce, Thai peanut sauce, or any other sauces you would like to have to spice up your meals.

I also recommend having a few frozen dishes on hand for emergencies, such as gluten-free fish sticks, frozen gluten-free bagels, gluten-free pasta meals such as macaroni and cheese or tuna noodle casserole, and so on. As you get used to the diet, you will find other things that you particularly enjoy and will want to keep those on hand at all times. Supplement with experimental choices and ingredients for new recipes. Your own kitchen is your refuge and your fallback for times when you are concerned about gluten contamination or just want to be confident that you always have something available to eat. Make sure it is well stocked with foods that bring you comfort and happiness.

Q: **If the package label says "manufactured in a facility that also produces wheat," is it still gluten-free?**

A: The answer is, it depends! Manufacturers now have to include that warning about the possibility of cross-contamination when it exists in their facility. The best thing to do is to contact the manufacturer directly and satisfy yourself that their cleaning and containment procedures are adequate to protect your safety.

Q: **Can I drink beer if I have celiac disease?**

A: Just a few short years ago, the answer was no. Thankfully, though, nationally and internationally distributed gluten-free beers are now available that do a tasty job of filling the beer void for celiacs. These manufacturers are using mixtures of such ingredients as sorghum and millet to produce gluten-free alternatives we can now enjoy. A few to look for include:

Redbridge Beer, from Anheuser-Busch
Green's beers, from Belgium
Hambleston ales, from England

Gluten-Free Baking Q&A

BELOW I have compiled a list of frequently asked questions by attendees in my cooking classes, consulting clients, and even professional chefs without a background in gluten-free and other food-allergy baking. Many of these questions are indeed "advanced," so do not worry if the thought never occurred to you to concern yourself with these details! Hopefully your questions will be addressed here as well.

Q: **How do you handle egg allergies when cooking gluten-free?**
A: Typical gluten-free recipes can often be adapted to utilize alternative products. Ener-G Egg Replacer is a well-respected substitute that works in most gluten-free recipes. Silken tofu, ground flaxseeds/flaxseed meal (approximately 1 tablespoon of flaxseed meal steeped for 10 minutes in $\frac{1}{4}$ cup boiling water), mashed bananas, pumpkin puree (approximately $\frac{1}{3}$ cup per egg being replaced), or 1 tablespoon unflavored gelatin to 1 cup boiling water—any of these options may work effectively to replace eggs in most recipes. Steer clear of trying to use egg substitutes in recipes where eggs make up a large portion of the ingredients, such as soufflés, angel food cakes, and omelets.

Q: **What if I need to eliminate both gluten and soy from my diet?**
A: Fortunately, many gluten-free recipes do not call for soy flour, and where they do, simply substituting an alternative grain such as sorghum does the trick. My all-purpose mix does not use any soy flour, so you can always fall back on that recipe or premixed flour. As far as other products go, just be vigilant about reading labels.

As for products based on soy—for example, many Asian sauces—it is hard enough to find these types of sauces without wheat, but add soy allergy to the mix, and finding a decent premade sauce for Asian foods becomes extremely difficult! Aside from using wonderful Thai peanut sauces (always check for wheat and soy ingredients, though!), try this easy homemade substitution instead: mix 1 tablespoon of molasses, 1/2 teaspoon rice vinegar, 1/4 teaspoon sea salt, 1/2 teaspoon sesame oil, and 1/4 cup gluten-free vegetable broth together in a small bowl. Whisk until blended. You can always make up a small container of your own sauce and carry it to your favorite restaurant. At least, that way, you'll be guaranteed to have a safe and delicious meal!

Q: **Many celiacs also have diabetes or precursors to diabetes that require a low-sugar diet. How do you make gluten-free foods with a low glycemic index?**

A: If you are gluten-free and cutting back on high-glycemic-index foods, try natural agave nectar in your baking. Agave nectar, an organic plant-based and unrefined sweetener, comes from the same agave plant that produces tequila. In addition to its wonderful sweetness, it has the advantage of offering a low glycemic index, which means it takes longer to be processed by the body and therefore causes less dramatic fluctuations in blood glucose and insulin levels.

You should also focus your recipe efforts on high-fiber whole-grain flours such as those discussed earlier in this appendix. Try to steer clear of a lot of simple carbohydrates such as white rice, white potatoes, and regular cane sugar.

To use agave nectar, pour it straight out of the bottle. It has a good shelf life of approximately three years and does not crystallize like honey, even when it is chilled. Light or amber agave nectars also make a perfect substitute for honey, and dark agave nectar works beautifully instead of molasses or maple syrup. For every cup of granulated cane sugar, use 3/4 cup agave nectar; however, expect to substitute agave cup for cup in recipes calling for liquids such as honey or molasses. When replacing granulated sugars with agave, reduce the other liquids in your recipe by approximately 1/4 to 1/3 cup for every cup of agave nectar used.

Q: **You say that gluten-free foods usually require additional leavening agents, so what do I use?**

A: In recipes calling for baking soda or baking powder, you will often add 50 to 75 percent more of that leavening agent in your gluten-free baked goods. Single-acting baking powders release carbon dioxide gas (the actual leavening agent) with the addition of moisture during the course of mixing the recipe. Thus, you want to put those recipes into the oven as soon as possible to avoid carbon dioxide loss.

I recommend using a double-acting baking powder in gluten-free baking because it will release some carbon dioxide when it becomes wet, but releases still more as it is heated in the baking process. You do not want to add too much of any leavening agent, though, as it could create too much carbon dioxide, which would disrupt the structure of your baked goods and force many gas bubbles to escape, causing the dough to collapse. Also be careful when increasing the amount of baking soda, as it can be bitter when used in excess. Baking soda works best when your recipe calls for acidic ingredients such as buttermilk, yogurt, sour cream, bananas, honey, or molasses, so be aware of other ingredients when deciding which leavening agents to add. Expandex Modified Tapioca Starch also helps to increase loft in gluten-free baked goods.

Q: What is the difference between potato flour and potato starch?

A: Potato starch is a very fine, bland tasting, white powder made by cooking peeled potatoes and dehydrating them to remove the starchy component. It is uncooked and thus does not absorb as much moisture from a recipe as does potato flour, which is cooked and is made from the whole potato, including the peel. The addition of the peel is probably the reason that potato flour has a slightly yellow patina in comparison to the potato starch. Potato starch is an excellent main ingredient in a gluten-free flour mixture, but potato flour may only be used in small amounts since it absorbs liquids so rapidly. If you put too much potato flour into a recipe, it will cause the food to be gummy; however, a little bit will be just sticky enough to help to hold a baked good together.

Q: What is the difference between rice flour and rice bran?

A: A grain of rice is made up of an outside kernel layer that contains bran and some rice germ. The bran contains the largest proportion of protein, antioxidants, and dietary fiber. It also contains a large amount of oil, which makes it more likely to turn rancid quickly if it is not heat treated before packaging or otherwise stored properly. "Polished rice" is rice from which the bran has been removed and is the component of rice from which rice flour is made. Sweet, white, and brown rice flours are all made from different polished rice grains.

Q: What is xanthan gum and what is guar gum?

A: Both xanthan and guar gums in their powdery form are useful substitutes for gluten when using gluten-free flour. Xanthan gum is created when a particular bacteria (*Xanthomonas campestris*) ferments with corn sugar to create a natural stabilizer or thickener with commercial uses in everything from ice cream (prevents ice crystals from forming) to salad dressings (acts as a stabilizer) to toothpaste (binds the paste to retain uniformity). It has widespread applications in gluten-free foods as well, since it replaces the stickiness of gluten that is so essential in holding foods together.[1] Guar gum is similarly useful, although naturally extracted from the guar bean. It has wonderful stabilizing qualities, increases dough yield, and improves the texture and shelf life of baked goods. It is sometimes used as a laxative due to its high soluble fiber content.[2]

Q: Are there other options besides xanthan or guar gum to use as binders in gluten-free flours?

A: Other options include using gelatin or pectin, applesauce, yogurt, dry milk or buttermilk powders. In a typical recipe, you should try ¼ cup applesauce, sour cream, yogurt, or dry milk powder per cup of gluten-free flour, or use 1 tablespoon gelatin.

---

1. Wisegeek, "What is Xanthan Gum," www.wisegeek.com/what-is-xanthan-gum.htm.

2. Wikipedia, "Guar Gum," http://en.wikipedia.org/wiki/Guar_gum.

Celiac Support Groups around the Country[1]

ALABAMA

Huntsville
North Alabama Gluten Intolerance Group
Contact: Jeana Swaim, President
Tel: (256) 233-8436
E-mail: jswaim@arilion.com

ALASKA

Anchorage
Celiac Sprue Association:
Contact: Michelle Johnson, State Coordinator
815 W. 12th Avenue
Anchorage, AK 99501
Tel: (907) 279-9856
E-mail: michelej@alaska.net

Anchorage Gluten Intolerance Group:
Contact: Alison L. Smith, Branch Manager
Tel: (907) 346-1405
E-mail: ancgig@customcpu.com

ARIZONA

Fountain Hills
Sunshine Chapter (CSA)
Contacts: Russ Boocock or Emma Teeter
16205 North Boulder Drive
Fountain Hills, AZ 85268-1519
Tel: (602) 837-1953 or (602) 820-5594

Green Valley
Contact: Kay Bleuer
E-mail: nkbleuer@yahoo.com

---

1. Adapted by permission of www.celiac.com. To access a similar list of regularly updated Raising Our Celiac Kids [ROCK] Groups, go to www.celiac.com/articles/226/1/ROCK-Raising-Our -Celiac-Kids–National-Celiac-Disease-Support-Group/Page1.html, or for a list of support groups outside of the United States, go to www.celiac.com/categories/Celiac-Disease-Support-Groups %2C-Organizations-%26-Contacts/Outside-the-USA%3A-Celiac-Disease-Support-Groups-and -Contacts/.

Payson

Payson Area Celiac Support Group
Contact: Nancy A. Palmer
HC 2 Box 95-S
Payson, AZ 85541
Tel: (520) 478-4383
Contact: Jane Kendall
HCR Box 305-B
Payson, AZ 85541
Tel: (520) 474-6707

Phoenix

Sunshine Celiac Support Group
Contact: Russ Boocock
16205 N. Boulder Drive
Fountain Hills, AZ 85268-1519
Tel: (602) 837-1953
Contact: Walter Koncar
1920 E. Inglewood Street
Mesa, AZ 85203

Phoenix

**Celiac Support of Greater Phoenix
(A CDF Connections Group)**
Contact: Diane Lake
Tel: (623) 587-8885
E-mail: dlake41@cox.net
Internet: www.phoenixceliac.com

Celiac Support of Greater Phoenix
Ruth Arieli
Tel: 480-922-7492
E-mail: arieliline@cox.net
Internet: www.phoenixceliac.com

Tucson

Southern AZ Celiac Support
Contact: Cheryl Wilson
11605 E. Golf Links Road
Tucson, AZ 85730
Tel: 520-298-5551
E-mail: rhranchaz@earthlink.net
Contact: Sue Beveridge
1807 W. Mountain Laurel Drive
Tucson, AZ 85737
E-mail: suebever@comcast.net

Contact: Jeannine Faidley
8479 East Tiffany Drive
Tucson, AZ 85715
Tel: (520) 298-9480
Internet: www.southernarizona
celiacsupport.org

ARKANSAS

Hot Springs Village

Contact: Betty Shepherd
11 Indiana Circle
Hot Springs Village, AR 71909
Tel: (501) 922-6034

Little Rock

Gluten-Free in Central Arkansas
Contact: Anne Luther
4710 Sam Peck Road, #1015
Little Rock, AR 72223
Tel: (501) 223-3981
E-mail: aaluther@comcast.net

Mountain Home

**Arkansas/Ozark Celiac Support
Group (CSA)**
Contact: Marilyn H. Jorgensen
198 Cochran Drive
Mountain Home, AR 72653
Tel: (501) 492-5243

Rogers

**Northwest Arkansas Celiac-Sprue
Group (Fayetteville, AR)**
Contact: Janice Carmichael
2703 Kathy Lane
Rogers, AR 72653-8725
Tel: (501) 636-8995

CALIFORNIA

Carlsbad

Contact: Helen Foreman
7112 Lantana Terrace
Carlsbad, CA 92011
Tel: (760) 931-7809
E-mail: bhforeman@webtv.net

Merced
Contact: Gary L. Brackney Sr.
3596 Hagen Court
Merced, CA 95348
Tel: (209) 722-7760

Modesto/Stockton/Turlock
Central Valley Celiacs
Contact: Karen Cadiz
Tel: (209) 823-3211
E-mail: centralvalleyceliacs@comcast.net

Newport Beach
Newport Beach Celiacs
Contact: Barbara Nielsen
440 Villa Point Drive
Newport Beach, CA 92660
Tel: (949) 644-4966
E-mail: glutenfreecoach@cox.net

Oakland
Sprue Group of the SF Bay Area
Contact: Ellen Switkes
116 Fairview Avenue
Piedmont, CA 94610
Tel: (510) 655-0215
E-mail: ellen@rutile.yi.org
Contact: Ellen Eagan
632 Miller Avenue
South San Francisco, CA 94080
Tel: (415) 583-6413
E-mail: eagan@pangloss.ucsf.edu

Orange County
Orange County Celiacs
Contact: Cecile Weed
Tel: (714) 750-9543

Palm Springs
Contact: Taylor Cushmore
2283 S. Alhambra Drive
Palm Springs, CA 92264
Tel: (760) 416-2051
E-mail: TaylorCush@aol.com

Redding
Contact: Karen Foss
795 Flower Ash Lane
Redding, CA 96003
Tel: (530) 222-1605

San Fernando Valley
San Fernando Celiacs (CDF Group)
Contact: Violla Orloff
Tel: (818) 345-8966

Sacramento
Sprue & You (CSA)
Contact: Diane Craig
Tel: (916) 483-8546
E-mail: dcraig101@hotmail.com
Contact: Kathleen G. Hughes
Tel: (530) 672-1104

San Bernardino
**Redlands Area Celiac Sprue
  Support Group**
Contact: Patricia Berger
627 Fountain Avenue
Redlands, CA 92373
Tel: (909) 793-3712
Contact: Robert V. Breunig
Highlander Hall Economics Dept.
University of California-Riverside
Riverside, CA 92521
E-mail: bbreunig@mail.ucr.edu

San Diego
**San Diego Celiac Sprue Association
  (CSA)**
Contact: Glorian Beeson
Tel: (760) 721-1791
E-mail: frankbeeson@cox.net
Contacts: William and Helen Foreman
7112 Lantana Terrace
Carlsbad, CA 92009
Tel: (760) 931-7809
E-mail: bhforeman@webtv.net
Contact: Sandy Milne
Tel: (858) 278-1413
E-mail: shipmates2@mindspring.com

San Rafael
Contact: Elizabeth Habberton
101 Pikes Peak Drive
San Rafael, CA 94903
Tel: (415) 472-4042

Santa Ana
Santa Ana Celiacs
Contact: Cecile Weed
13471 Marty Lane
Garden Grove, CA 92843
Tel: (714) 750-9543
Contact: Debbie Lee
Tel: (714) 830-8237

Santa Cruz
Santa Cruz Celiac Support Group
Contact: Pam Newbury
543 Ice Cream Grade
Santa Cruz, CA 95060
Tel: (831) 423-6904
E-mail: pknewbury@earthlink.net

Santa Rosa
Sonoma County CSA
Contact: Laura Southworth
480 Bohemian Highway
Freestone, CA 95472
Tel: (714) 798-3112
Contact: Rosemary Yates
129 Grenvillia Drive
Petaluma, CA 94952
Tel: (707) 766-8606

Stanford
Stanford Celiacs
Contact: Kelly Rohlfs
Stanford University
Palo Alto, CA 94305
Tel: (650) 725-4771
E-mail: krohlfs@stanford.edu

Stockton
Central Valley Celiacs (CSA)
Contact: Karen Cadiz

E-mail: centralvalleyceliacs@comcast.net
Tel: (209) 823-3211

Temecula
Contact: Arlene Gibbs
42013 Thoroughbred Lane
Murrieta, CA 92562
Tel: (909) 696-9730

Ventura County
Ventura County Celiacs
Contact: Kathy Button
2525 Waxwing Avenue
Ventura, CA 93003
Tel: (805) 650-0520
E-mail: venturaceliac@sbcglobal.net
Internet: www.venturaceliac.org

COLORADO

Berthoud
Contact: William R. Eyl
2600 Blue Mountain Avenue
Berthoud, CO 80513
Tel: (303) 772-3155

Colorado Springs
Pikes Peak (CSA)
Contact: Virginia Ludwig
3705 Meadowland Boulevard
Colorado Springs, CO 80918
Tel: (719) 598-6748
Contact: Therese Stock
Tel: (719) 442-0422

Denver
Denver Celiac Sprue Association (CSA)
Contact: Betty Elofson
Tel: (303) 238-5145

Denver
Denver Celiacs, Denver Metro Area
Contact: Donna Steelman
4617 S. Joplin Way
Auroa, CO 80015
Tel: (303) 699-6170

E-mail: donnasteelman@comcast.net
Contact: Jill Smith
2289 W. Hyacinth Road
Highlands Ranch, CO 80216
Tel: (303) 683-3281

Fort Collins
Northern Colorado Chapter (CSA)
Contact: Deborah Fusco
4610 Shoreline Road
Fort Collins, CO 80526
Tel: (970) 226-4105
E-mail: dfusco@hach.com
Contact: Delores Valdez-Amick
803 S. Van Buren Avenue
Loveland, CO 80538
Tel: (970) 663-4048

Highlands Ranch
Contact: Mary Ann Peterson
10111 S. Silver Maple Road
Highlands Ranch, CO 80126
Tel: (303) 683-1461

CONNECTICUT

Danbury/Waterbury
Nutmeg Chapter (CSA)
Contact: Suzel Cable
548 High Street, 2nd Floor
Naugatuck, CT 06770
Tel: (203) 723-1318
Contact: Edith K. Meffley
Tel: (203) 438-6108

Glastonbury
Contact: Beth Hillson
262 Cedar Ridge Drive
Glastonbury, CT 06033
E-mail: beth@glutenfree.com

Hartford
Greater Hartford Area Chapter (CSA)
Contacts: Edward and Dorothy
    Corcoran
39 Glenwood Road

South Windsor, CT 06074
Tel: (860) 644-1335

Milford
**Greater New Haven Celiac
    Children's Group**
Contact: Pat Vlamis, Cochair
26 Cheryl Lane
Prospect, CT 06712
Tel: (203) 758-0106
E-mail: pmazz@snet.net

New Haven
Greater New Haven Celiac Group
Contact: Bill Jacobs
100 Alexander Drive
Cheshire, CT 06410
E-mail: wajacobs15@aol.com

Northwest Connecticut
**Celiac Support Group of Northwest
    Connecticut (CSA)**
Contact: Marilyn Duffany
Tel: (203) 283-8506

Suffield
Celiac Discussion Group
Contact: Kathy Bosse
PO Box 307
Suffield, CT 06078
Tel: (860) 668-4835
E-mail: Kathybosse@aol.com

Waterbury/Nutmeg
**Celiac Sprue Support Group of
    NW Connecticut**
Contact: Carol Hoebel
84 Woodruff Avenue
Thomaston, CT 06787
Tel: (860) 283-5577
E-mail: david.hobel@snet.net
Contact: Suzel Cable
548 High Street, 2nd Floor
Naugatuk, CT 06770
Tel: (203) 723-1318

Contact: Edith K. Meffley
Tel: (203) 438-6108
Contact: Joan Balough
Tel: (203) 268-3829
Contact: Syd Aronowitz
Tel: (203) 794-0150

DELAWARE

Wilmington/Newark
Delaware Celiac and Gluten Intolerant Group—New Castle County
Contact: Eva Szalewicz
Tel: (302) 482-4882
E-mail: gluten-free@yahoogroups.com

DISTRICT OF COLUMBIA

Washington, D.C.
Washington Area Celiac Support Group
Contact: Juanita Ohanian
Tel: (301) 881-4018
E-mail: jaonebel@aol.com
Internet: www.dcceliacs.com

FLORIDA

Clearwater
Pinellas County Celiac Group(CSA/USA Chapter #84)
Contact: Jim and Mary DuGranrut
St. Petersburg/Clearwater, FL
Tel: (727) 522-1204
E-mail: jdug@pipeline.com

Crystal River
Crystal River Celiacs
Contact: Mary Lou Thomas
6350 W. Patriot Street
Homosassa, FL 34448
Tel: (352) 628-9559
E-mail: mlthomas4cs@hotmail.com

Melbourne
GIG of Florida
Contact: Mary Kump

3190 Village Park
Melbourne, FL 32934-8296
Tel: (407) 254-2034
Contact: Michael Jones
E-mail: mjones@digital.net

Naples
Contact: Barbara Rattigan
2500 Kings Lake Boulevard
Naples, FL 34112
Tel: (941) 775-7747

Orlando
Celiacs of Orlando
Contact: Michael Jones
12733 Newfield Drive
Orlando, FL 32837
Tel: (407) 856-3754
E-mail: mjones@digital.net

Palm Beach
Palm Beach County Celiac Support Group
Contact: Phyllis Kessler
15927 Laurel Creek Drive
Delray Beach, FL 33446
Tel: (561) 637-0396

Pensacola
Contact: Nancy Kilpatrick
5433 Lee St. West
Milton, FL 32570
Tel: (904) 626-0064

Sarasota
Sarasota Celiacs
Contact: Edith Kaplan
E-mail: ediesrq@verizon.net
Internet: www.sarasotamanateeceliacs
.com

Tampa Bay
Tampa Bay Celiacs
Contact: Janet Heitler
8106 North Albany
Tampa, FL 33604

Tel: (813) 933-1645
E-mail: jchtbc42@tampabay.rr.com

GEORGIA

Savannah
The Savannah Celiac Support Group (GIG)
Contact: Nancy Wheeler, Branch Manager
11 Ale House Retreat
Savannah, GA 31411
E-mail: ncwheelee@yahoo.com

Smyrna-Support Group
Atlantic Celiac Support Group (CSA)
Contact: Jan Austin
Tel: (404) 433-9661

Atlanta
The Gluten-Sensitive Support Group
Contact: Bernie Mercer
Tel: (404) 728-1508
Fax: (404) 728-9491

IDAHO

Boise
Boise Idaho Celiac Support Group
Contact: Twylia McIlvanie
Tel: (208) 939-0373
E-mail: Scott Neil-SNeil@Cableone.net

North Idaho
Contact: Jeanne Dickson
1303 W. Longhorn Road
Rathdrum, ID 83858
Tel: (208) 687-8225
E-mail: gfjeanne@msn.com

ILLINOIS

Champaign
Champaign-Urbana Celiac Support Group
Contact: Tammy Frick

702 Devon Drive
St. Joseph, IL 61873
Tel: (217) 469-7674
E-mail: GF911@AOL.COM

Chicago
Celiac Sprue Association of Greater Chicago
PO Box 93
Arlington Heights, IL 60006
Tel: (847) 255-4156
Internet: www.csagc.cjb.net

Decatur
Contact: Jewell M. Barr
3333 Lost Bridge Road
Decatur, IL 62521
Tel: (217) 423-8234

Joliet
Contact: Jenn Cain
303 Rivers Edge Drive
Minooka, IL 60447
E-mail: jacsgroup@sbcglobal.net

Marseilles
Illinois Valley Celiac Group
Contact: Sherri J. Mathews
2631 E. U.S. Highway 6
Marseilles, IL 61341
Tel: (815) 795-4260
E-mail: dmathews@bb-elec.com

Peoria
Central Illinois Celiacs (CSA)
Contact: Marsha Bishoff
619 Spring Street
Washington, IL 61571
Tel: (309) 444-7415 or (309) 692-3848
Contact: Pat Weinkauf
825 West Meadows Place
Peoria, IL 61604
Contact: Kate Jowick
E-mail: Kate_Joswick@ccmail.wiu.edu

Petersburg
Land of Lincoln Celiac
Support Group
Contact: Barb Hand
RR 3, Box 276C
Petersburg, IL 62675
Tel: (217) 632-2684

Rockford
Rockford Area Chapter (CSA)
Contact: Jolyn M. Fasula
6816 Crown Ridge
Rockford, IL 61103
Tel: (815) 877-5302
Contact: Ron Ford
Tel: (815) 229-8804

INDIANA

Bloomington
Contact: Roberta Rezits
1908 Arden Drive
Bloomington, IN 47401
Tel: (812) 332-6454

Evansville
Evansville Celiac Sprue Support
Group
Contact: Barbara Watson
1317 Bayard Park Drive
Evansville, IN 47714
Contact: Gloria Baker
2711 Knob Hill Drive
Evansville, IN 47711
Tel: (812) 476-5744

Indianapolis
Celiac Support Group of Indianapolis
(CSA)
Contact: Joyce Etheridge
1168 Sheffield Drive
Avon, IN 46123
Tel: (317) 272-4609
E-mail: mjbetheridge@aol.com
Contact: Diane Hosek
1371 Stoney Creek Circle

Carmel, IN 46032
Tel: (317) 569-9670
E-mail: dianehosek@gmail.com

Lafayette
Indiana Gluten Intolerance
Support Team (CSA)
Contact: Nancy H. Linnemann
2635 N 400 W.
West Lafayette, IN 47906
Tel: (765) 497-0665
E-mail: n.linnemann@insightbb.com

La Porte
Contact: Margaret M. Diffendorfer
1012 Wright Avenue
La Porte, IN 46350
Tel: (219) 362-6607

IOWA

Carroll
Contact: Lynne Humphrey
121 S. Maple Street
Carroll, IA 51401-3123
Tel: (712) 792-5866
E-mail: hump@win-4-u.net

Cedar Rapids
Cedar Rapids Support Group
(CRCC GIG)
Contact: Theresa Brandon
2407 Linwood Street S.W.
Cedar Rapids, Iowa 52404-3554
Tel: (319) 362-8087
E-mail: tatbrandon@gmail.com
Internet: www.iowaceliacs.org

Davenport
Quad City Celiac Group
Contact: Becky Wentworth
6130 N. Hancock Avenue
Davenport, IA 52806
Tel: (563) 391-2968
E-mail: wentworth@netexpress.net

Iowa City

Iowa City Celiacs
Contact: Sarah Berke
735 Michael Street, #32
Iowa City, IA 52246
Tel: (319) 337-9521

Manchester

N.E.I. Celiacs Support Group
Contact: Marcia Intorf, President
307 Gay Street
Delhi, IA 52223
Tel: (563) 922-2470
E-mail: msintorf@fbx.com
Contact: Lynn Cooper, Secretary
923 Doctor Street
Manchester, IA 52057
Tel: (563) 927-3870
E-mail: 923dlcoop@n-connect.net

Tipton

**Living Free Celiac Disease
    Support Group**
Contact: Jacey Drollinger
Tipton, IA 52772
Tel: (319) 886-6255

Waverly

Eastern Iowa Celiacs
Contact: Jill Everding
Denver, IA 50622
Tel: (319) 984-5928
E-mail: everding@forbin.net
Contact: Brenda Whiteside
Shell Rock, IA 50670
Tel: (319) 885-6680
E-mail: whiteside@netins.net

Waterloo

Waterloo and Cedar Falls Celiacs
Contact: Kristi Simmerman
1753 Robin Road
Waterloo, IA 50701
Tel: (319) 234-2104
E-mail: simmerman@bigfoot.com

KANSAS

Kansas City

Greater Kansas City Celiacs (CSA)
Contact: Helen Richards
14409 W. 123rd Terrace
Olathe, KS 66062
Tel: (913) 393-2400
E-mail: richgary@swbell.net
Contact: Karen and Roger Miller
11714 Hadley
Overland Park, KS 66210
Contact: Danelle Sorensen
Olathe, KS
Tel: (913) 397-9284
E-mail: homesweethome@yahoo.com

Leavenworth

Contact: Latisha May Thomas
1313 Vilas
Leavenworth, KS 66048
Tel: (913) 682-6678

Manhattan

Manhattan Celiac Support Group
Contact: René Eichem
2442 Buttonwood Drive
Manhattan, KS 66502
Tel: (913) 776-6013
Contact: Mary Jordan
2513 Nutmeg
Manhattan, KS 66502
Tel: (913) 539-2963
E-mail: MJordan672@aol.com

Topeka

**Topeka Celiac Sprue Support Group
    (CSA)**
Contact: Sharon Larson, President
4310 SE McMahan Court
Tecumseh, KS 66542
Tel: (785) 379-0479
E-mail: slars5@cox.net

Wichita
Wichita Celiacs (CSA)
Contact: Kay Finn
805 N. Cypress
Wichita, KS 67206
Tel: (316) 686-7034
Internet: www2.southwind.net/
~weeks/celiac/

KENTUCKY

Benton
Heartland CS.DH of W. KY/S. IL
Contact: Rose Mary Mueller
102 Wyndy Brook Lane
Benton, KY 42025
Tel: (270) 527-8330
E-mail: heartlandceliac@bellsouth.net
Internet: www.heartlandgig.org

Louisville
Greater Louisville CS Support Group
Contact: Marge Johannemann
5622 Elmer Lane
Louisville, KY 40214-4781
Tel: (502) 368-6338
Contact: LaVaughan Will
2104 Northfield Drive
Louisville, KY 40222
Tel: (502) 425-3561
E-mail: lvhwill@aol.com
Contact: Rebecca Smith-Ritchey
2 11 W. Oak Street, #1015
Louisville, KY 40203
Tel: (502) 562-1778

LOUISIANA

Baton Rouge
Celiacs of Baton Rouge
Contact: Mary Mack-Jeansonne,
President
3387 Madeira Drive
Baton Rouge, LA 70810
Tel: (225) 766-8872
E-mail: celiacsbr@aol.com

New Orleans
**Greater New Orleans Celiac Sprue
Support Group**
Contact: Diane Schaefer
Tel: (504) 348-3099
Contact: Lorraine McCaslin
Tel: (504) 833-1717

American Celiac Society
Contact: Annette Bentley, President
PO Box 23455
New Orleans, LA 70183-0455
Tel: (504) 737-3293
Internet: www.americanceliacsociety.org

Slidell
Contact: Jamie Head
3771 Arrowhead Dr.
Slidell, LA 70458
Tel: (504) 643-2676

MAINE

Bangor
**Celiac Sprue Support Group of the
Greater Bangor Area**
Contact: Ann Delaware
PO Box 472
Bradley, ME 04411-0472
Tel: (207) 827-2733
Contact: Greg Chappelle
27 Hilliard Street
Old Town, ME 04468
25 Cushing Drive
Glenburn, ME 04401-1431
Tel: (207) 947-9958

Bradley
Bradley Celiacs
Contact: Ann Delaware
PO Box 472
Bradley, ME 04411
E-mail: Anned0472@aol.com

Portland

**Portland Maine Celiac/DH
Support Group (CSA)**
Contact: Paula Raleigh
130 Kimball Corner Road
Naples, ME 04055
Tel: (207) 787-2279
E-mail: honeybee@pivot.net

MARYLAND

Annapolis

Chesapeake Celiac Support Group
Contact: Patricia Minnigh
(410) 672-5834
Internet: www.celiacsonline.com

Baltimore

Maryland Chapter (CSA)
Contact: Phyllis Farmer
600 Straffan Drive, Unit 502
Timonium, MD 21093
Tel: (410) 560-1279
Contact: Doug Rettberg
498 South Hills Court
Westminster, MD 21158
Tel: (410) 876-3604

Bethesda

**Montgomery County Support Group
Washington Area Celiac Support
Group**
Contact: Juanita Ohanian
Tel: (301) 881-4018
E-mail: jaonebel@aol.com
Internet: www.dcceliacs.com

Delmarva

**Maryland Delmarva Celiac Support
Group**
Contact: Betty Bellarin
E-mail: bbrboc@comcast.net

MASSACHUSETTS

Boston

**Children's Hospital-GI/Nutrition
Dept.**
300 Longwood Avenue
Boston, MA 02115
Tel: (617) 355-2127
E-mail: celiacsupportgroup@childrens
.harvard.edu

**The Healthy Villi-Greater Boston
Celiac/DH Support Group (CSA)**
Contact: Lee Graham, Chairperson
E-mail: randlgraham@comcast.net
Contact: Catherine Mirick
Membership Chairperson
Tel: 888-4-CELIAC
Internet: www.heathyvilli.org

Cape Cod

Cape Cod Support Group
Contact: Diane Bertrand
PO Box 1114
North Falmouth, MA 02556
E-mail: DMBertrand@adelphia.net
Contact: Margo Finnell
E-mail: Margo820@juno.com

Fall River

**Southeast New England (including
Cape Cod) Celiac Support Group**
Contact: Kathy Thiboutot
Tel: (401) 624-8888

Lowell

Contact: Katherine C. Merrill
45 Tolman Avenue
Lowell, MA 01854
Tel: (978) 454-2822

MICHIGAN

Ann Arbor

Gluten-Free Ann Arbor
Contact: Valerie Mates

E-mail: gfaa@unixmama.com
Internet: health.groups.yahoo.com/
  group/GlutenFreeAnnArbor/

Antrim and Kalkaska County
Contact: Linda Bicum
Tel: (231) 322-2811

Benzie County
Contact: Betty Robotham
Tel: (231) 325-5725

Coldwater
Contact: Bruce and Ruth Young
335 Barnhart Road
Coldwater, MI 49036
Tel: (517) 278-8248

Dryden
Tri-County Celiac Support Group,
  SE Michigan
Spru-Nik Press
Contact: Robin Donagrandi
21580 Birchwood
Farmington, MI 48336
Tel: 86-NOGLUTEN
E-mail: TCCSG@twmi.rr.com
Internet: www.tccsg.com

Escanaba
Contact: David A. Jondrow
312 Minneapolis Avenue
Gladstone, MI 49837
Tel: (906) 428-1621

Flint
Mid-Michigan Celiacs
Contact: Nyla E. Wilson
11029 Phyllis Drive
Clio, MI 48420
Tel: (810) 686-2539

Gladstone
Contact: David A. Jondrow
312 Minneapolis Avenue

Gladstone, MI 49837
Tel: (906) 428-1621

Grand Rapids
West Michigan Celiac Support Group
Contact: Mitzi J. Berkhout
753 Parkway Drive NE
Grand Rapids, MI 49505
Tel: (616) 363-5749
Contact: Sue Baker
686 Carpenter NW
Grand Rapids, MI 49504
Tel: (616) 691-4906
Contact: Rosalynn Hausman
E-mail: mwhausman@aol.com

Kalamazoo
CSA of Greater Kalamazoo
Contact: Annette Hensley
Tel: (269) 492-5278
Contact: Michelle Rutan
Tel: (269) 342-1533

Lansing
Contact: Greta DeWolf
1815 Sandhill Road
Mason, MI 48854
Tel: (517) 349-0294
Internet: micapitalceliacs.atspace.com

Mid-Michigan Chapter (CSA)
Contact: Donovan J. Sprick
Tel: (313) 733-6857

Traverse City
Traverse Area Gluten-Free Support
  Group (TAGFSG)
Contact: Sandra Cartwright
PO Box 4112
Traverse City, MI 49685-4112
Tel: (231) 947-8324
E-mail: Scarttc@aol.com
Contact: Kathy DiMercurio
Tel: (231) 946-1687
Contact: Kelli Sefton (children)
Tel: (231) 943-0878

MINNESOTA

Brainerd Lakes Area
Contact: Jennifer Chock
Brainerd, MN
Tel: (218) 825-9525

Grand Rapids
Range Area Celiac Support Group
Contact: Angeline Edgar
Tel: (218) 328-5731
E-mail: rangeceliac@yahoo.com

Minneapolis/St. Paul Area
**Northland Celiac Support Group
(formerly Midwest Gluten
Intolerance Group)**
Contact: Carol Hansen
Tel: (651) 489-0645
E-mail: carolahansen@comcast.net
Contact: Barbara Wojcik
Tel: (651) 653-4523
E-mail: barbara1760@comcast.net
Internet: www.northlandceliacs.org

Rochester
**Southeast Minnesota Celiac Support
Group**
Contact: Coyla Shepard, Founder
2805 Hidden Hills Lane NE
Rochester, MN 55906
Contact: Warren Budd
Tel: (507) 288-9056

MISSISSIPPI

Gulfport
Mississippi Celiac Support Group
Contact: Jane Dacey
PO Box 1276
Ocean Springs, MS 39566
Tel: (601) 875-2820

MISSOURI

Branson
Tri Lakes Celiac Support Group
Contact: Barbara Hicks

9 Arrowhead Road
Kimberling City, MO 65686
Tel: (417) 739-2703
E-mail: honedu@centurytel.net

Columbia
**Columbia MO Gluten-Free Support
Group**
Contact: Donna Kasper
Columbia, MO 65203
Tel: (573) 447-5659
E-mail: n2kasper@mchsi.com

Kansas City
Contact: Elanor R. Aadams
135 N. Missouri
Liberty, MO 64068
Tel: (816) 781-6514

Saint Louis
Saint Louis Chapter (CSA)
Contact: Bill Vellios Sr.
812 Kehrs Mill Road
Ballwin, MO 63011-2442
Tel: (314) 391-6855
Contact: Joan Fitzsimmon
6716 Westway Road
St. Louis, MO 63109
Tel: (314) 351-5114
Contact: Linda Ritter
E-mail: nltr@charter.net

MONTANA

Alzada
Contact: Teri Lindberg
HC 56, PO Box 60
Alzada, MT 59311

Big Timber
Contact: Debra Barrett
PO Box 1018
513 W. Third
Big Timber, MT 59011

Billings
Contact: Dennis McGough
1023 Marie Dr.

Billings, MT 59101
Tel: (406) 256-5569

Bozeman/Helena
Montana Celiac Society
Contact: R. Jean Powell
1019 S Bozeman Avenue, #3
Bozeman, MT 59715
Tel: (406) 586-1285
E-mail: rjeanp@aol.com

Chester
Contact: Ruth Wardell
PO Box 251
Chester, MT 59522
Tel: (406) 759-5874

Choteau
Contact: Jeanette Rasmussen
4210 Highway 89
Choteau, MT 59422
Tel: (406) 466-2091

Columbus
Contact: Jeanne Murray
PO Box 594
Absarokee, MT 59001-0594
Tel: (406) 328-4851

Deer Lodge
Contact: Eloise Faber
911 Missouri Avenue
Deer Lodge, MT 59722
Tel: (406) 846-1246

Helena
Contact: Cleo Anderson
PO Box 4637
Helena, MT 59604
Tel: (406) 227-6671
E-mail: cleomt@aol.com
Contact: Judy Harris
1817 Silver Street
Helena, MT 59601
Tel: (406) 443-5158

Missoula
Contact: Dottie Caluori
1440 River Street
Missoula, MT 59801
Tel: (406) 542-7499

Wolf Point
Contact: Alice Whitmer
872 Nickwall Road
Wolf Point, MT 59201
Tel: (406) 525-3289

NEBRASKA

Grand Island
Central Nebraska Celiacs
Contact: Keith McTavish
PO Box 411
Wood River, NE 68883
Tel: (308) 583-2949

Grand Island
Contact: Diane D. Epp
Box 595
Henderson, NE 68371
Tel: (402) 723-4759

Lincoln
Star City Area Chapter (CSA)
Contact: Beckee Moreland
1639 Sunset Road
Lincoln, NE 68506
Tel: (402) 441-9621
E-mail: beckland@inebraska.com

Omaha
Omaha Chapter (CSA)
Contact: Mary A. Schluckebier
PO Box 31700
Omaha, NE 68131-0700
Tel: (402) 558-0600
E-mail: csaceliacs@csaceliacs.org

Midlands Chapter (CSA)
Contact: Lynn Samuel
6303 Kentucky Road
Papillion, NE 68133

Tel: (402) 339-1346
Contact: Rebecca Warren
Tel: (402) 235-3576

Seward

Contact: Mary Schluckebier
1616 Plainview Avenue
Seward, NE 68434
Tel: (402) 643-4340

NEVADA

Las Vegas-Resource:
Contact: Joanne B. Mathews
270 W. Basic Road
Henderson, NV 89015

Las Vegas

Contact: Catherine Hammelrath
3355 Rolan Court
Las Vegas, NV 89121
Tel: (702) 733-7633
E-mail: vegascat53@cox.net

Reno

Reno Celiacs & Nutrition Resources
Contact: Kerry Seymour
475 Hill Street, Suite C
Reno, NV 89501
Tel: (775) 329-8811

NEW HAMPSHIRE

Laconia

Contact: Ann Marie Shumway
31 Havenwood Drive
Laconia, NH 03246
Tel: (603) 528-1911

Nashua Area

Contact: John Waksmonski
Tel: (603) 437-1702
Contact: Christine Muir
E-mail: themuirs@charter.net

Portsmouth

Contact: Dan Davis
6 Oakridge Road

Kensington, NH 03833
Tel: (603) 778-1938
E-mail: djdavis107@comcast.net

NEW JERSEY

Brick
Contact: Gary Powers
284 White Oak Court
Brick, NJ 08724
Tel: (732) 840-3718

Cherry Hill

Contact: Fran Twersky
107 East Burgess Road
Marlton, NJ 08053-1202
Tel: (609) 983-3362

Hackettstown

Contact: Mrs. Merle Morse
PO Box 148
Hackettstown, NJ 07840
Tel: (908) 852-7311

Long Branch

Specialized Pediatric Celiac Group
Specialized Ped. Ambulatory Center
307 3rd Avenue
Long Branch, NJ 07740
Tel: (201) 870-5216

Maple Shade

Contact: Cindy Fisher
377 Crawford Avenue
Maple Shade, NJ 08052
Tel: (856) 779-1562
E-mail: hfishernj@aol.com

New Brunswick

Celiac/DH Support Group and
    Cel-Kids Network (CSA)
Contact: Diane Eve Paley
22 Island Drive
Old Bridge, NJ 08857-2518
Tel: (908) 679-6566
E-mail: DEPaley@AOL.COM
Contact: Alex Schwedack

5-C Twin Rivers Drive
East Windsor, NJ 08520
Tel: (609) 443-6623
Contact: Rosanna Beck
Tel: (908) 225-7594
E-mail: B6724@aol.com

Old Bridge
**Central Jersey Celiac/DH Support
Group (CSA)**
Contact: Diane Eve Paley
22 Island Drive
Old Bridge, NJ 08857
Tel: (732) 679-6566
E-mail: DEPaley@aol.com

Paramus
**American Celiac Society-Bergen
County**
Contact: Lauri Schlussel
11 Marz Road
Westwood, NJ 07675-8217
Tel: (201) 573-0397

Princeton
Contact: Evelyn Sasmor
Tel: (609) 279-0770
E-mail: evelyn@sasmor.com

South Jersey
Southern New Jersey Chapter (CSA)
Contact: Bill Lucas, Chairperson
330 Saint Mary Street
Burlington, NJ 08016
Tel: (609) 387-7139
E-mail: lucaswe@earthlink.net
Contact: Leah Edelstein,
Cochairperson
23 Stevens Drive
Voorhees, NJ 08043
Tel: (856) 435-6785
E-mail: ledelstein@comcast.net
Contact: Patti Townsend,
Cochairperson, Membership
Collingswood, NJ

Tel: (856) 854-5508
E-Mail: tompatti@comcast.net

NEW MEXICO
Albuquerque
**Albuquerque Gluten Intolerance
Support Group**
Celiac Sprue Association-New Mexico
Contact: Marilyn Johnson, State
Coordinator
Tel: (505) 299-5283
E-mail: marilynyj@comcast.net

Las Cruces
Las Cruces Celiacs
Contact: Susan Pieper
4825 Senita
Las Cruces, NM 88011
Tel: (505) 522-8182
E-mail: spieper@huntel.com

NEW YORK
Albany
**Capital District Celiac Support Group
(Albany-ACS)**
Contact: Katie Marschilok
4 Fairlawn Lane
Troy, NY 12180
Tel: (518) 271-1784
E-mail: Marschilok@aol.com
Contact: Barbara Jordan
Tel: (518) 439-8652

Batavia
Contact: Virginia R. Baldwin
PO Box 158
Pavilion, NY 14525
Tel: (716) 584-3422

Binghamton
Celiac Self-Help Group
Contact: Nancy Dorfman
12 Laurel Avenue
Binghamton, NY 13905
Tel: (607) 722-3848

Buffalo

Gluten-Free in WNY (GIG)
Contact: Mike Lodico
PO Box 24
N. Tonawanda, NY 14120
Tel: (716) 694-3287
E-mail: glutenfree2@gmail.com
Contact: Joanne Hameister
Tel: (716) 655-0849
E-mail: jeham@buffnet.net
Internet: www.glutenfreeinwny.com/

Ithaca/Cornell

Contact: Laura Johnson-Kelly
48 Comfort Road
Ithaca, NY 14850
Tel: (607) 272-5902
E-mail: LWJ1@cornell.edu
Contact: Mary Ochs
18 Whig Street
Trumansburg, NY 14886
Tel: (607) 387-9221
E-mail: mao4@cornell.edu

Long Island

Long Island Celiacs
Contact: JoanAnn Defiglia
1023 Jackson Avenue
Franklin Square, NY 11010
Tel: (516) 437-0396
Contact: Ellen Mulligan
193 5th Street
Hicksville, NY 11801
Contact: James J. Callahan
Tel: (516) 794-1654

Middletown

Celiac Kids' Club
Contact: Marisa Frederick
264 Scotchtown Road
Goshen, NY 10924
Tel: (914) 294-1385

Mohawk Valley

The Celiac Support Group of the Mohawk Valley
(Chapter of Celiac Disease Foundation)
Contact: Eleanor P. Wallace
10 Clinton Street, Apt. 715
Whitesboro, NY 13492
Tel: (315) 736-6981
E-mail: elpar6@yahoo.com
Internet: www.csgmv.org/

New Paltz

Mid-Hudson Valley Gluten-Free Outings Meet-Up Group
Contact: Tovah
E-mail: glutenfreebay@gmail.com
Tel: (845) 255-0671

New York City

Greater New York Celiac Support Group (CSA)
Contact: Mary Ferry
Tel: (212) 304-1026
Contact: Merle Cachia
Tel: (212) 662-2464
E-mail: pjc1@columbia.edu

Plattsburgh

North Country Celiac Support Group
Contact: Shirley Koester
Tel: (518) 643-9461
E-mail: redwing2@localnet.com

Rochester

Rochester Celiac Support Group
Contact: Susan Kath
1039 Moseley Road
Fairport, NY 14450
Tel: (585) 425-9994
Contact: Marvin Becker
210 Crandon Way
Rochester, NY 14618
Tel: (585) 442-9528

E-mail: www.rochesterceliacs.org/
contact.htm
Internet: www.rochesterceliacs.org

Suffolk County
Suffolk County Celiacs (GIG)
Contact: Les Doti
PO Box 13
Kings Park, NY 11754-0013
Contact: Michael Thorn
Tel: (631) 395-5071
E-mail: SuffolkCeliacs@aol.com
Internet: www.suffolkcountyceliacs.org

Syracuse
**Central New York Celiac Support
Group**
Contact: Ruth Wyman
263 Roxbury Road
Syracuse, NY 13206
Tel: (315) 463-4616
E-mail: jwyman1@twcny.rr.com

White Plains
**Westchester Celiac Sprue
Support Group**
Contact: Chris Spreitzer
PO Box 66
Montrose, NY 10548-0066
Tel: (914) 737-5291
E-mail: info@westchesterceliacs.org
Contact: Lou Zimet
E-mail: louzimet@optonline.net

Williamsville
**Western NY Gluten-Free Diet
Support Group (CSA)**
Contact: Cliff Hauck, Cochairperson
PO Box 1835
Williamsville, NY 14231
Tel: (716) 636-6021
E-mail: hauckc@adelphia.net
Internet: www.buffaloglutenfree.org

NORTH CAROLINA

Asheville
Contact: Leah R. Karpen
518 Ox Creek Road
Weaverville, NC 28787
Tel: (704) 645-9067

Boone
Contact: Ernest Lane
827 Blairmont Dr.
Boone, NC 28607
Tel: (704) 264-4618 or
(704) 262-2380
E-mail: epl@math.appstate.edu

Charlotte
Charlotte Celiac Support Group
Contact: Caroline Herdle
14314 Harbor Estates Road
Charlotte, NC 28278
Tel: (704) 588-6842
E-mail: Katahdin1@pipeline.com
Contact: Daphne Ledford
2037 Meadowood Lane
Charlotte, NC 28211
Tel: (704) 366-3493
E-mail: DFLedford@aol.com

Durham-Fayetteville
North Carolina Celiacs (CSA)
Contact: Ruth Thomas
Tel: (919) 542-4030
Contact: Susan Black
Tel: (910) 875-3186

Raleigh-Durham
Triangle Celiac Support Group
Contact: Diana Clarke
E-mail: DeBucket@aol.com
Contact: Connie Margolin
E-mail: ThirdEar0@aol.com

NORTH DAKOTA

Bismarck
Central ND Celiac Resource Group
Contact: Lila Brendel
1900 93 Street SE
Bismarck, ND 58504
Tel: (701) 258-7800
E-mail: CNDC_GIG@msn.com

Oakes
North Dakota Celiacs (CSA)
Contact: Juli Becker
10585 85th Street SE
Oakes, ND 58474
Tel: (701) 742-2738

OHIO

Canton
Alliance Area Celiac Support Group
Contact: Denise Ramey
Tel: (330) 966-1515
E-mail: daramey33@netzero.net

Cincinnati
Cincinnati Celiac Support Group
Contact: Denise Ramey
Children's Hospital Medical Center
Cincinnati, OH 45229
Tel: (513) 887-7153
E-mail: president@cinciceliac.com
Internet: www.cinciceliac.com

Cleveland
Northeast Ohio Celiac Support Group
Contact: Trisha Lyons
2500 MetroHealth Drive
Cleveland, OH 44109
Tel: (216) 778-7835
E-mail: TLyons@metrohealth.org
E-mail: Clevelandceliac@yahoo.com
Internet: www.geocities.com/
  clevelandceliac/

Greater Cleveland Celiac Association (CSA)
Contact: Cindy Koller-Kass, President
33040 Rockford Drive
Solon, OH 44139
Tel: (440) 248-6671
E-mail: glutenfree1@yahoo.com

Columbus
Gluten-Free Gang
Contact: Mary Kay Sharrett
700 Children Drive
Columbus, OH 43205-2696
Tel: (614) 722-3093
E-mail: sharretm@chi.osu.edu
Contact: Monica Hrabowy
663 Laurel Ridge Drive
Gahanna, OH 43230
Tel: (614) 337-1833
E-mail: EHrabowy@aol.com
Internet: www.glutenfreegang.org

Dayton
**Miami Valley Celiac Sprue
  Support Group**
Contact: Sandra Leonard
560 Park Hills Crossing
Fairborn, OH 45324
Tel: (513) 878-3221
E-mail: thebaker30@sbcglobal.net
Contact: Barbara Wieland
5903 S. Tecumseh Road
Springfield, OH 45502
Tel: (937) 324-8652
E-mail: wielandbj@aol.com

Mansfield
**Richland County Celiac
  Support Group**
Contact: Bev Messner
First Presbyterian Church
399 S. Trimble Road
Mansfield, OH
Tel: (419) 589-5972
E-mail: bevmessner@aol.com
Internet: www.rccsg.com

Toledo

Contact: Daniel and Linda Judson
147 West Front Street
Perrysburg, OH 43551
Tel: (419) 874-2519
Contact: Jean Meagley
620 Sawyer Road
Toledo, OH 436156
Tel: (419) 578-4947
E-mail: CattyGranny@aol.com
Internet: http://glutenfreesupportof
toledo.com

OKLAHOMA

Norman

Contact: Kate Martin
Norman, OK
Tel: (405) 364-5612
E-mail: one4life@swbell.net
Internet: http://katesceliac.blogspot.com

Oklahoma City

**Oklahoma Celiac Sprue Support
Group (CSA)**
Contact: Heather Cline
1403 Classen Drive, Oklahoma City,
OK 73106
Tel: (405) 235-1715
E-mail: HMCline@aol.com
Internet: www.OKceliac.com

Okmulgee

Contact: Barbara Sipple
Rt. 1, Box 247
Morris, OK 74445
Tel: (918) 733-4571

Tulsa

Celiac Sprue Association, Tulsa Chapter
Contact: Ronda Falkensten
St. Francis Education Resource Building
St. Francis Hospital
6161 S. Yale Avenue
Tulsa, OK 74136
E-mail: info@csatulsa.org

OREGON

Bend

**Central Oregon Gluten Intolerance
Group (GIG)**
Contact: Lynelle Thomas
2442 NW Marken
Bend, OR 97701
Tel: (541) 389-1731

Burns

Contact: Nici Bailey
449 S. Diamond
Burns, OR 97720
Tel: (541) 573-1164

Portland/Vancouver

Portland Metro GIG Branch
Contact: Mary Wikle, Branch Manager
PO Box 4204
Tualatin, OR 97062-4204
Tel: (503) 692-0724
E-mail: mwikle_carousel@yahoo.com

Salem

Contact: Ann Grafe
1328 Dogwood Drive
Woodburn OR 97071
Tel: (503) 982-3644

PENNSYLVANIA

Bethlehem (Allentown area)

Contact: Carla Madden
809 Race Street
Catasauqua PA 18032
E-mail: kapanagia@yahoo.com

Danville

ACS Danville City Support Group
Contact: Elaine M. Jeffreys
RD 6 Box 143C
Danville, PA 17821
Tel: (717) 275-0654

Carroll Valley

Gluten-Free Group of Gettysburg
Contact: Cheryl Hutchinson
22 Ski Run Trail
Carroll Valley, PA 17320-8537
E-mail: hutchjc@earthlink.net

Harrisburg

GIG of Harrisburg
Contact: Linda L. Weller
PO Box 312
Hershey, PA 17033
Tel: (717) 520-9817
E-mail: Harrisburg@gluten.net
Internet: www.harrisburgceliacs.org

Indiana

**Indiana Regional Medical Center
Celiac Support Group**
Contact: Brenda Shilling,
    Director of NFS
Indiana Regional Medical Center
Indiana, PA 15701
E-mail: bshilling@indianarmc.org

Lancaster

Lancaster Area Celiacs
George and Becky Maag
Tel: (717) 367-9257
E-mail: lancasterareaceliacs@yahoo.com
Internet: www.lancasterareaceliacs.org

Mount Pleasant

Mount Pleasant Celiac Support Group
Contact: Vicky Vrabel
616 West Main Street
Mount Pleasant, PA 15666
Tel: (724) 542-9745

Philadelphia

ACS Whoo Sprue Group
Contact: Laura Sposito
1211 Tree Street
Philadelphia, PA 19148
Tel: (215) 336-5004

**Greater Philadelphia Area Celiac
Sprue Support Group**
Contact: Karen Dalrymple
583 Valley View Road
Langhorne, PA 19047

Pittsburgh

**Pittsburgh East Area Celiac
Sprue Support**
Contact: Elsie Janthey
204 George Lane
Pittsburgh, PA 15235
Tel: (412) 823-2010
Contact: Lois Kosoglow
Tel: (412) 744-2356
Contact: Ruth Masengill
Tel: (412) 327-5564

**Greater Pittsburgh Celiac Sprue
Support Group (CSA)**
Contact: Lorraine Weaver,
    Treasurer and Membership
1446 Greenbriar Court
Library, PA 15129
Tel: (412) 835-4983 or (412) 833-9507
Contact: Theresa Fogle
Tel: (724) 335-4892
E-mail: tfogle1@aol.com

State College

**Central Pennsylvania Celiac Support
Group**
Contact: Cindy Sunderland
RD 2, Box 189
McVeytown, PA 17051-9618
Tel: (717) 899-6482
E-mail ras@dd1.arl.psu.edu

Wilkes-Barre/Scranton

**Wilkes-Barre/Scranton Celiac
Support Group (CSA)**
Contact: Pattie Kupetz
17 W. Sunrise Drive
Pittston, PA 18640
Tel: (570) 602-7459

Wynnewood
Contact: Rita M. Herskovitz
52 Rockglen Road
Wynnewood, PA 19096
Tel: (215) 642-9351

York
Gluten-Free Health Group
Contact: Kathie Cavanagh
18 Valley Road
Jacobus, PA 17407
Tel: (717) 428-3859
E-mail: kcavanagh@wellspan.org

RHODE ISLAND

Providence
**MA & RI Celiac Support Group
for Children**
Contact: Tanis Collard
11 Level Acres Road
Attleboro, MA 02703-6843
Tel: (508) 399-6229
Internet: http://members.home.net/
kellyleech/celiac/csgc.html

**American Celiac Family Support
Group of RI**
Contact: Linda Monahan
155 Reservoir Road
Pascoag, RI 02859
Tel: (401) 568-6110
E-mail: MonahanLinda@yahoo.com
Internet: www.celiacsupportgroup.com

SOUTH CAROLINA

Columbia
Palmetto Celiac Support Group
Contact: Peggy Smith
1508 Anthony Drive
West Columbia, SC 29172
Tel: (803) 775-9466 or (803) 755-7291

Florence
Contact: Lea E. Marshall
1214 Hillside Avenue
Florence, SC 29505
Tel: (803) 665-6290

TENNESSEE

Jackson
Contact: Allan Clement
151 Lone Oak Drive
Jackson, TN 38305
Tel: (731) 423-5315
E-mail: aclementhome@hotmail.com

Knoxville
Contact: Theresa Cornelius
7424 Oaken Drive
Knoxville, TN 38938-4321
Tel: (865) 922-8780
E-mail: TheresaCornelius
@Changing-Lifestyles.com

Memphis
Memphis Area Celiac Support Group
Contact: Lisa Trenthem
1753 Carruthers Place
Memphis, TN 38112
Tel: (901) 276-7751
E-mail: ltrenthem@utmem.edu
Contact: Sally Damron
E-mail: srdamron@bellsouth.net

Nashville
**Nashville Celiac Support Group
(CSA)**
Contact: Christine Fry
E-mail: cfry@comcast.net
Tel: (615) 837-0875
Contact: Janet Lowery, Newsletter
E-mail: janetlowery@comcast.net
Tel: (615) 758-7967
Contact: Maureen Norris, Treasurer
E-mail: manorris@comcast.net
Tel: (615) 591-9616

TEXAS

Austin

Alamo Celiac Austin Gluten Intolerance Group
Contact: Francie Kelley
Tel: (512) 301-2224
E-mail: fkelley@austin.rr.com
Internet: www.alamoceliac.org

Austin Gluten-Free Friends
Contact: Kay Stence
5604 Southwest Parkway, #3113
Austin, TX 78735
Tel: (512) 442-4008
E-mail: kstence@marykay.com

Brazoria County

Brazoria County Texas Celiac Support Group
Contact: Cecilia McNeil
Tel: (979) 265 0819
E-mail: clmcneil@academicplanet.com

Corpus Christi

Alamo Celiac Corpus Christi
Contact: Susan M. Revier, Secretary
Tel: (361) 855-6810
E-mail: jamesrevier@grandecom.net

Dallas

Lone Star Celiac Gluten Intolerance Group
Contact: Sandy Klein, President
1600 Aldridge Drive
Plano, TX 75075
Tel: (972) 424-2307
E-mail: sandyklein1@comcast.net
Internet: http:www.dfwceliac.org

Eastland

Contact: Jill Hollywood
PO Box 938
Eastland, TX 76448-0938
Tel: (254) 629-1299

Fort Worth

North Texas Gluten Intolerance Group
Contact: Betty Barfield, President
6821 Nob Hill Drive
North Richland Hills, TX 76180
Tel: (817) 967-2804
E-mail: betty.barfield@aa.com
Internet: www.northtexasgig.com

Houston

Houston Celiac Sprue Association
Contact: Janet Y. Rinehart, Chairman
13722 Ashley Run
Houston, TX 77077
Tel: (281) 679-7608
E-mail: txjanet@swbell.net
Internet: http://www.houstonceliacs.org

Lubbock

Lubbock Celiac Support Group
Contact: Rebecca Holland
Internet: http://www.lubbockceliac group.com

Midland

West Texas GF Awareness Group
Contact: Pat Gatlin
11809 W. County Road, #54
Midland, TX 79707
Tel: (915) 563-4847
Contact: Lois Newbold
Tel: (915) 684-4671
Contact: Linda Blanchard
E-mail: linda@ccgs.com

San Antonio

Alamo Celiac San Antonio
Contact: Anne Barfield
606 Jackson Keller
San Antonio TX 78216-7121
Tel: (210) 340-0648
E-mail: AnneBarfield@satx.rr.com
Contact: Lynn Rainwater
1023 Cloverbrook

San Antonio TX 78245-1604
Tel: (210) 673-3041
E-mail: txlynnr@swbell.net

Texarkana
Contact: Marie Freeman
Rt 6, Box 465-F
Texarkana, TX 75501
Tel: (903) 793-1392

UTAH

Statewide
Gluten Intolerance Support
Groups of Utah
Internet: www.gfutah.org

Northern Utah
Celiac Support Group of
Northern Utah (GIG)
Contact: Marie Kawaguchi
E-mail: mkawag@msn.com
Tel: (801) 732-9363

Salt Lake City
Salt Lake Gluten Intolerance Group
(GIG)
Contact: Pam Ward, Sandi Bigelow,
Tim Coda, Cochairs
Contact: Marcie Coda, Branch
Manager
St. Mark's Hospital (meeting place)
E-mail: saltlakegig@gmail.com
Internet: www.gfutah.org

Utah County
Contact: Paul Faris
Tel: (801) 225-5828
E-mail: pfaris@juno.com

Utah County Gluten Intolerance
Group (GIG)
Contact: Robert and Amber Lee
Tel: (801) 763-0977
E-mail: info@gfutah.org
Internet: www.gfutah.org

VERMONT

Bennington
Southern Vermont Celiacs
Contact: Lynn Grieger
RD 3 Box 586
Arlington, VT 05250
Tel: (802) 375-9069

St. Albans
Celiac Support Group of Vermont
Contact: Suzanne Ludlam
E-mail: rsludlam@yahoo.com

VIRGINIA

Alexandria
Washington Area Celiac Support
Group
Contact: Juanita Ohanian
Tel: (301) 881-4018
Fax: (301) 230-1970
E-mail: jaonebel@aol.com
Internet: www.dcceliacs.com

Blacksburg
New River Valley CS Support Group
Contact: John Tice
Blacksburg, VA
Tel: (540) 951-2126
E-mail: jtice1@johntice.com

Charlottesville
Celiac Sprue Support Group
Contact: Amy E. Pagano
Tel: (434) 243-4666

WASHINGTON

Aberdeen/Hoquiam
Gluten Intolerance Group of
Grays Harbor
Contact: Julie Evensen
Contact: Kris Morrison, RN
E-mail: gigofgraysharbor@yahoo.com

Bellingham
Bellingham Gluten Intolerance Group
Contact: Kelle Rankin-Sunter
Tel: (360) 332-7435
E-mail: info@glutenfreeway.info
Internet: www.glutenfreeway.info

Centralia
Lewis County Area Gluten
   Intolerance Group
Contact: Sam Jennings
Tel: (360) 385-2282
E-mail: cybersam13@msn.com

Ellensburg
Ellensburg Gluten Intolerance Group
Contact: Jamie Macke, Branch
   Manager
Tel: (509) 859-3780
E-mail: glutenfree@charter.net

Olympia
Olympia Gluten Intolerance
   Support Group
Contact: Eve Brown
Tel: (360) 493-7507
E-mail: evelyn.brown@providence.org
Contact: Joe Spancic
Tel: (253) 964-0299
E-mail: jkspancic@comcast.net

Port Townsend
Port Townsend Gluten
   Intolerance Group
Contact Adele Fosser
Tel: (360) 385-2282
E-mail: fosserha@olypen.com

Seattle
Central Seattle Group
Contact: Steve Wangen, ND
Tel: (206) 264-1111
E-mail: info@ibstreatmentcenter.com
Internet: www.ibstreatmentcenter.com/
   7–c.htm

SnoKing Celiac Support Group
Contact: Sue Corning
Tel: (206) 527-6678
E-mail: penguinea@hotmail.com

Seattle/Bellevue/Renton
Seattle Celiacs
Contact: Earl Ley
Tel: (425) 747-1110
E-mail: earl.ley@comcast.net
Internet: www.seattleceliacs.com

Sequim
Kitsap/Olympic Peninsula
   Gluten Intolerance Group
Contact: Susan Eliot
Tel: (360) 477-4548
E-mail: seliot@wavecable.com

Vancouver
Gluten Intolerance Group of
   SW Washington
Contact: Kristi Curtis
Tel: (360) 695-0862
E-mail: justus323@yahoo.com
Internet: www.gigsouthwestwa.org

Walla Walla
Blue Mountain Gluten Intolerance
   Group
Contact: Evelyn Bergman
Tel: (509) 522-2053
E-mail: hjbneab@charter.net

Whidbey Island
Whidbey Island GIG
Contacts: Coyla Shepard and
   Sydney Anderson
Tel (Coyla): (360) 321-4083
Tel (Sydney): (360) 321-4272
E-mail: coylajohn@whidbey.com
Internet: www.gigbranches.org/
   whidbeyisland

WEST VIRGINIA

Hurricane
West Virginia Gluten Intolerance
Group
Contact: Karen Daniel
Tel: (304) 757-0696
E-mail: krdaniel@suddenlink.net
Internet: www.orgsiges.com/wv/wvgig

Acknowledgments

MANY THANKS to all those who have helped me in my own
gluten-free journey to good health and happiness. My parents, in particular, have offered me seemingly limitless encouragement and love,
and for that I will be eternally grateful. Many dear friends have happily tasted not only my successful gluten-free recipes but also my early
and singularly untasty experiments as well. These honest tasters helped
me strive for a better way to cook gluten-free. Without these willing
subjects (many of whom no doubt sacrificed a pants size in the process), I would never have known how my recipes compare to wheat-
flour recipes. So, for that assistance, we can all be grateful.

In addition to such tasting assistance, I am blessed by many friends
like Jack and Mary Stansbury, Monique and Warren Burke, and Laura
and Dave Thurston, who have overlooked how consumed I have been
with this book in recent months and have nonetheless happily invited
me to their tables. Holly Dawsey's sage counsel kept me sane, and
their collective friendship and love have been my daily source of
strength.

Dr. Alessio Fasano and his team at the University of Maryland
Center for Celiac Research, in particular Pam King, Maggie Burk, and
Pam Cureton, have proven invaluable to me over the years. They
never tire of spreading awareness of celiac disease and have supported

my efforts from the very beginning. Knowing them all now as friends, I appreciate even more their honest dedication to teaching about, healing, and one day preventing celiac disease. Dr. Fasano remains one of the busiest people I know, yet he nonetheless dedicated precious time to give thoughtful attention to reviewing and writing the foreword to this book.

To all of those who write me with your woes, your questions, your successes, and your struggles with celiac disease, thank you for not settling for mediocre gluten-free foods or mundane gluten-free lives. Appreciative words and evocative questions from such companions have inspired me to tackle new kitchen challenges and have guided much of the content of this book. To those whom I have met in my gluten-free journey who have generously agreed to share their personal stories, I thank you each for enhancing the richness of information conveyed to the readers by allowing me to use your words to describe your own lives with celiac disease. I must especially acknowledge the efforts, time, and energy Chrissy Andrews devoted to this book and to the larger cause of helping others with celiac disease to live nearly normal lives again.

I am grateful to Dr. Monique Burke for agreeing to take precious moments away from her newborn daughter to describe in layman's terms pediatric protocols regarding celiac testing and recommending gluten-free diets for children. Thanks also to my dear friend Gabrielle Jacobson for the countless hours she no doubt spent skillfully editing the bulk of this manuscript. Tracey Thompson's ever-poignant suggestions, even though made from a distance of hundreds of miles away, found their way into the text and content and doubtless made it a better book, just as she has made me a better person over these many years of friendship. Jeff Rasmussen's late-night reviewing and prose suggestions carried me through many rounds of edits and his gift of tunes helped me type into the wee hours with a smile.

I cannot fail to recognize Glenna Patrick and all of my wonderful Catonsville friends (Laura, Mary, Monique, Debbie, Annie, Jill, Laurie, Kathy, Anne, Terry, Sandi, Mimi, Nina . . .) who enabled me to complete this book on schedule, as they each pitched in to entertain and care for my children at various times. I suppose in some circumstances, it does take a village to write a book!

My agent, Marilyn Allen, deserves much credit for having the vision to see me in the role as teacher for others learning to live gluten-free after a diagnosis with celiac disease. She never doubted that I was the right one for this job.

Finally, I would like to give due credit to my editor, Katie McHugh, and those others at DaCapo Press who had the foresight to recognize the need for such a book dedicated to celiac disease. The content and formatting guidelines they devised lend unique clarity to the subject for the newly diagnosed as well as for those who have been struggling to live well with celiac disease.

Index